Food & Fitness *after* 50

Eat Well, Move Well, Be Well

CHRISTINE ROSENBLOOM
PHD, RDN, FAND

BOB MURRAY
PHD, FACSM

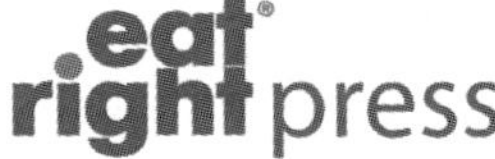

Academy of Nutrition and Dietetics
CHICAGO, IL

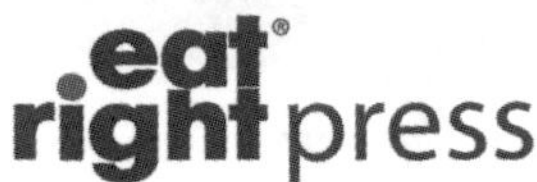

Academy of Nutrition and Dietetics
120 S. Riverside Plaza, Suite 2190
Chicago, IL 60606

Food and Fitness After 50: Eat Well, Move Well, Be Well

ISBN 978-0-88091-956-2 (print)
ISBN 978-0-88091-957-9 (eBook)
Catalog Number 956218 (print)
Catalog Number 956218e (eBook)

The views expressed in this publication are those of the authors and do not necessarily reflect policies and/or official positions of the Academy of Nutrition and Dietetics. Mention of product names in this publication does not constitute endorsement by the authors or the Academy of Nutrition and Dietetics. The Academy of Nutrition and Dietetics disclaims responsibility for the application of the information contained herein.

10 9 8 7 6 5 4 3 2 1

For more information on the Academy of Nutrition and Dietetics, visit www.eatright.org.

Library of Congress Cataloging-in-Publication Data

Names: Rosenbloom, Christine, 1951- author.
Title: Food and Fitness After 50 : Eat Well, Move Well, Be Well / Christine Rosenbloom, PhD, RDN, FAND, Bob Murray, PhD, FACSM.
Other titles: Food and Fitness After Fifty
Description: Chicago, IL : Academy of Nutrition and Dietetics, [2018] | Includes bibliographical references and index.
Identifiers: LCCN 2017036887 (print) | LCCN 2017043321 (ebook) | ISBN 9780880919579 (eBook) | ISBN 9780880919562 (print)
Subjects: LCSH: Older people--Nutrition--Popular works. | Exercise for older people. | Older people--Health and hygiene.
Classification: LCC RA777.6 (ebook) | LCC RA777.6.R665 2018 (print) | DDC 613.7/10846--dc23
LC record available at https://lccn.loc.gov/2017036887

To those over 50 who want to eat well, move well, be well...
and feel younger than your age.

TABLE OF CONTENTS

ABOUT THE AUTHORS

Christine (Chris) Rosenbloom, PhD, RDN, FAND, wanted to be a dietitian since she was 13 years old. Under her picture in her North Olmsted, OH, high school yearbook is the title Future Dietitian. After a college degree in nutrition at Kent State University and a dietetic internship at the University of Minnesota, she became a registered dietitian nutritionist and worked as a clinical dietitian in Atlanta area hospitals. She joined the faculty of nutrition at Georgia State University in 1980, where she taught nutrition for 30 years. Her doctoral studies focused on sociology with a concentration in gerontology.

Currently, Chris is a nutrition professor emerita and runs a small business providing nutrition consulting services to many food and nutrition-related groups. She has more than 40 years of experience in nutrition, with specialties in sports nutrition and gerontology. For more than 25 years, Chris has provided nutrition advice to athletes of all ages. And teaching health professionals and gerontology students about health and aging motivated her to pay attention to her own aging. She has always enjoyed with working with active people, and her academic experience in gerontology led to the desire to combine the two—sports nutrition and aging—into a book about food and fitness for those over 50.

Chris and her husband, Rob, live on Lake Hartwell, GA, where they enjoy entertaining friends and family, spending time with their 37 nieces and nephews. Chris is a recreational athlete who enjoys swimming, cycling, kayaking, golfing, hiking, walking the dogs, and taking aerobics and yoga classes at the local YMCA.

Robert (Bob) Murray, PhD, FACSM, never intended to become an exercise physiologist. When faced with the decision of choosing a college major, Bob opted for his favorite class in high school—gym class. After receiving his master's degree in physical education, Bob was fortunate to land a job as an assistant professor of health and physical education, along with being a men's swimming and diving coach, at Oswego State University on the shores of Lake Ontario in upstate New York. Three years later, Bob realized it was time for more education because his swimmers kept asking him questions about nutrition and training that he couldn't answer. In the mid-70s, one of the top exercise-physiology programs in the country was at Ohio State, so Bob continued his education there, graduating with a PhD in 1980.

Armed with his doctorate, Bob set out to continue his career as a college professor and was hired at Boise State University, where he spent the next five years working, living, and playing in the great city of Boise. In the spring of 1985, a single phone call changed Bob's life and career path. The Gatorade Company was looking for an exercise physiologist to start an internal research laboratory to help support the business. Then part of the Quaker Oats Company based in Chicago, the Gatorade business was founded on scientific research conducted at the University of Florida, and Gatorade executives wanted to continue that reliance on science. Bob served as director of the Gatorade Sports Science Institute (GSSI) from 1985 to 2008, leading a team of exercise and nutrition scientists, external advisors, and researchers to develop the wide-ranging scientific and education offerings of GSSI, a truly unique enterprise in a corporate setting. Research conducted by Bob and his team on the hydration needs of athletes and physiological and performance responses to fluid, carbohydrate, and electrolyte ingestion has contributed to the broader understanding of the importance of being well hydrated during exercise and of the role that carbohydrate and electrolytes play in helping athletes and nonathletes alike get the most out of their bodies during physical activity.

Bob is now managing principal of Sports Science Insights, LLC, a consulting group that assists companies and organizations in need of targeted expertise in exercise science and sports nutrition. Sports Science Insights's clients range from start-ups to Fortune 100 companies. Bob is a fellow of the American College of Sports Medicine and an honorary member of the Academy of Nutrition and Dietetics.

FOREWORD

YOU MIGHT THINK it's presumptuous for an old, beat-up football player and coach to write a foreword for a nutrition book. I have a confession to make: I'm as passionate about food as I am about fitness.

My passion for food and fitness began at a very young age. My father was four decades ahead of his time in nutrition and weight training. We had plenty of green vegetables, protein powder, and pure yogurt at our house in 1948. Proper food and physical training were a religion for us, and, subsequently, I have always assumed no one could teach me anything I didn't already know on the subject.

When my friend, Christine Rosenbloom, PhD, RDN, FAND, asked if I could write a foreword for her book, I wasn't sure I would learn anything new. I thought this book would be touting more of the stuff I have known for decades. But I am delighted to admit that I could not have been more wrong!

Rosenbloom and Murray have done a masterful job of pulling together reams of information for aging adults on this crucial subject, analyzing and personalizing it, and then relating the vital principles in a concise, fun to read style. In every chapter, they describe a real person in their 50s, 60s, 70s and beyond who embodies and humanizes their principles. There is a very good chance that you will find yourself in one of these "real life stories."

In the introduction, the authors list five C's as a foundation for the book's approach: Clarity of information, Confronting the myths, Confidence to make choices, Consistency in actions, and Concise recommendations, all utilized to reach a sixth C: Control over your health and well-being.

After reading this book, I suggest there is a hidden seventh C that captures the essence of their work for me, a lifelong nutrition enthusiast, and this is Consolidation. Throughout the book, the authors reinforce and synthesize complex information into clear and actionable advice on eating and exercise. In your hands, you have a resource that is brief but thorough, scientific but fun, and organized without tedium. It literally consolidates all we need to know to eat well, keep moving, and have energy and good health in our second half of life.

Way to go Chris and Bob!

Bill Curry

Former NFL starting Center for the Super Bowl champion Green Bay Packers (Super Bowl I and II)

Retired College Football Coach (Georgia State University, University of Kentucky, University of Alabama, Georgia Institute of Technology)

ESPN College Football Analyst

Speaker, Author, Motivator

ACKNOWLEDGMENTS

WE WANT TO thank many people, but we specifically want to extend our gratitude to the following:

Thank you to the many people who embraced the book's concept and helped us get started by providing questions and comments in focus groups, at community lectures, through many individual conversations, and through our webpage surveys. Sharing your personal stories of successes and challenges as you've aged helped shape the book and make it real.

Our gratitude goes out to the experts quoted in our "Conversation with an Expert" sections. These friends and colleagues, who are all over the age of 50, freely gave of their time to lend insight into how they eat well, move well, and be well by translating their research into actionable steps.

We also want to thank the Publications, Resources, and Products team at the Academy of Nutrition and Dietetics, who provided leadership and guidance through the entire process of writing the book.

We want to recognize the four talented experts in nutrition, exercise, and aging who shared their expertise and insights to strengthen the final work: Lisa Carlson, MS, RDN; Robin B. Dahm, BS, BA, RDN, LDN; Mary Ellen Posthauer, RDN, LD, CD, FAND; Marianne Smith Edge, MS, RDN, LD, FADA.

Lastly, we would not be here without our patient and supportive spouses, Rob Rosenbloom and Linda D'Ambrosio Murray, who have always been our biggest champions. We appreciate all of your support.

INTRODUCTION

Stephanie has been dieting for most of her life. A few years before her 50th birthday, she turned to comfort foods to help her escape the stress of caring for aging and ill parents, a demanding professional career, no work-life balance, and little free time. She knew she should exercise, but her motivation was zapped. But then she teamed up with a friend, and they started walking a few times a week during lunchtime. She found that walking helped her feel better. The friends decided to have a friendly competition to motivate each other to lose weight. Stephanie lost some weight, but what really clicked was the realization that activity not only helped her lose weight but also helped her de-stress and clear her head. Walking became her go-to activity. As her birthday loomed, Stephanie was grieving the recent death of her mother and was spread thin by the demands of continuing to care for her father. Because there were so many things going on in her life that she couldn't control, Stephanie realized that she needed to figure out what she could control and what would help her feel happier. She decided that she could be "fit and 50"; her age wasn't under her control, but her food and fitness choices were.

LIKE STEPHANIE, WE often feel that so many things in life are beyond our control, but what we eat and our level of fitness are often under our control. Each day, we face lots of decisions about what to eat, when to eat, and how active we should be. For many of us, the default mode is to choose the easy path. After all, it is easier to make reservations than to make dinner or to binge-watch our favorite television show instead of going to the gym. We rationalize our choices by saying, "it's in my genes," or "it's too late for me to change," or "it's too complicated," or "I don't have time," or "I'm exhausted. Maybe I'll start tomorrow," or "it happens as we age." Complicating matters is the perception that nutrition and fitness advice seems so controversial and ever changing.

We want to share this book with you because we know firsthand that a common-sense approach to food and fitness leads to active, healthy life that can be balanced with a rewarding career or happier retirement. We are increasingly dismayed by the nonsense that regularly appears in popular diet books, blogs, magazines, and online sources. We see poorly qualified people lecture about how to eat, what foods to buy, how to exercise, and how to stop the aging process (wouldn't that be nice?). This book will translate competent scientific research into simple, actionable steps. Our approach is simple, and you will learn what it takes to control your food choices and fitness strategies as you navigate your 50s, 60s, 70s, and beyond. This is not a textbook; it goes beyond lecturing about nutrition and fitness information and answers your questions with effective tools and real-life strategies you can use to maintain and enhance your health.

Each section of this book will arm you with the five Cs needed to help you reach the sixth and most important C—*Control*:

Clarity of science to understand the hows and whys of food and fitness,

Confronting the myths by untangling common food and fitness myths,

Confidence to choose healthy foods and the best exercise strategies to see real changes,

Consistency of advice to help you quickly find the most relevant information, and

Concise information to help you hone in on the most critical information.

Each chapter also includes:

- the bottom line up front so that you can quickly understand the key message of each chapter;
- stories from individuals who want to achieve fitness and choose healthy foods but look for shortcuts or strategies that miss the target they seek—these case studies illustrate how you can avoid the same pitfalls;
- self-assessments that can help you honestly assess your food and fitness decisions; you can use the assessments to encourage you to keep up the good work and nudge you toward improving your nutrition and health;
- questions older adults commonly ask about many health and nutrition topics;
- conversations with nutrition and fitness experts from around the globe to help you understand in clear and simple terms how to stay fit and eat well; and
- tips from the authors on how they eat healthy and stay physically active.

The book is divided into three sections: Eat Well, Move Well, and Be Well. In each section, the normal aging process will be used to anchor the recommendations. After all, what we ate and drank and how we stayed fit in our 20s and 30s likely won't meet our needs in our 50s and beyond.

In the Eat Well section, we will focus on healthy dietary patterns and the food choices that can give you the right balance of nutrients. We will shift the focus from dead-end thinking on topics such as good carbs or bad fats to making common sense choices about foods that will give your body the nutrients it needs for good health and fitness. Our advice will not include counting fat grams or worrying about sugar calories. Instead, we shift the focus to making the right decisions about the foods you love. We will dispel such myths as "never eat white foods," "sugar is toxic," or "bacon is bad." You will learn how to choose the best protein foods, whether you are a Paleo lover or a vegetarian, and how to distribute protein throughout the day to protect your muscle mass. This section also includes hydration plans and the best beverage choices for health and fitness. No Eat Well section would be complete without taking a look at alcohol and the latest science related to health and longevity. This section also goes beyond food and drink to help you decide if you need vitamin, mineral, or other dietary supplements and how to make safe, effective choices.

In the Move Well section, we'll examine all dimensions of fitness, from preserving strength and building muscle to enhancing endurance and maintaining balance. Whether you have been inactive for decades or are already dedicated to fitness, we'll help you choose activities that improve your strength, cardiovascular fitness, and flexibility. Some adults believe you can't build strength and muscle after 50, but that is not so. In a landmark study in 1994, researchers showed that even among sedentary, elderly nursing home residents, muscle strength was improved by regular resistance exercise, and enhanced muscle strength improves walking gait and balance, reducing the risk of falls.

In the Be Well section, we put it all together—how to eat the foods you like to support your body weight and fitness goals. While not a diet book, this is a food-and-fitness book that can help with weight loss, weight maintenance, or weight gain. The information and advice in this book will give you a personalized road map to get healthy and stay healthy. Many other things impact our ability to be well: sleep quality, social interactions, stress reduction, mindfulness, and laughter all help us be our best selves at any age.

It is never too late to eat right and exercise the smart way. You can be healthier and more fit in your 60s than you were in your 40s; chronological age is not a determinant of functional age. But we are not naive; even with the best eating habits and smart exercise plans, stuff happens. Active adults do sometimes need joint replacement surgery. "Use it or lose it" is a frequent theme for aging body parts, but so is "abuse it and lose it." Joint problems, broken bones, and cancer afflict even the healthiest among us. Good nutrition and fitness can reduce the risk of chronic disease, but even active adults get high blood pressure, diabetes, or heart disease. None of those things need deter you from the path of good health—and some might even be the motivator you need to take control. Sure, it might slow you down, refocus your goals, or change your exercise routine, but most of us who are lucky enough to be in older age demographics ultimately face health challenges. Instead of complaining or worrying about getting older, we should be mindful that not everyone gets the privilege of long life. So instead of complaining, we should take control.

Read, reflect, and rely on our expertise to help you get on a good path to healthy, enjoyable eating and engaging physical activity. Accept the challenge, make a change, and connect with us on your path to good health. We will come back to visit Stephanie in the book's epilgoue to see how she took control of her food and fitness, so stay tuned!

CHAPTER

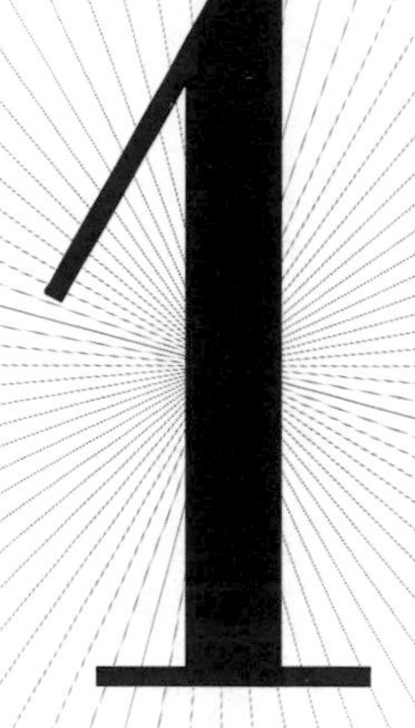

HOW TO GET STARTED ON A FOOD AND FITNESS AFTER 50 JOURNEY

The Bottom Line

To eat healthy and be fit over age 50 doesn't require the latest diet book, a 3-hour daily grueling workout, or supplements that claim to burn fat and speed metabolism. With some tweaks to your usual diet and by making a commitment to a physical activity plan, you can be healthier at 65 than you were at 45. Consider the 100-year-old woman who broke the 80-years-and-over world record for the 100-yard dash at the 122nd Penn Relays in Philadelphia. She didn't start exercising until she was 67 years old, proving that it is never too late to get started. Here are a few things to keep in mind about health, fitness, and aging:

- **The body experiences many changes with age, but it is hard to separate normal aging from disease and usual aging from the disuse of a sedentary lifestyle.**
- **Monitoring body weight and tracking physical activity can provide motivation to eat better and get fit, but no one way works best for everyone.**
- **Eating for optimal aging can include many different healthy eating patterns; one size does not fit all.**
- **Physical activity may be the best thing you can do to "use it" instead of losing it. Along with preventing or slowing loss, you can actually improve muscle tone, bone density, metabolism, and even cognitive function with physical activity.**

At age 30, Susan, who is 5 feet 4 inches, weighed 125 pounds and had a body mass index (BMI) of 21.45—a healthy weight with a low risk of cardiovascular disease and diabetes according to statistics. Fast forward 30 years and Susan weighs 185 pounds and has a BMI of 31.75, putting her in the obese category. She also has high blood pressure and elevated cholesterol. How did it happen? Weight creep. Susan never monitored her weight and gained a couple of pounds every year. At first, 2 pounds doesn't seem like a lot, but multiply 2 pounds by 30 years and you're saddled with a 60-pound weight gain.

Tony, a three-sport high school athlete and college soccer player thought his active youth and early adult years would confer lifelong benefits. Today, at age 58, he gets winded walking up a couple of flights of stairs. While his weight hasn't changed much, his body composition has. More fat and less muscle has left him with prediabetes, and if he doesn't make some lifestyle changes, things will get worse.

Introduction

Most adults over age 50 know they should eat better and exercise. In fact, retirees say that health, not wealth, is the number one ingredient for happiness as they age. Let's face it: food tastes good, and exercise requires effort. However, we will show that you can still enjoy favorite foods and include physical activity to move to a healthier place. How many adults can say they are in the best health in their 50s and beyond? Unfortunately, the numbers don't lie.

- Among older American adults, 30% are overweight or obese.
- Only one in five American adults meets the recommendations for daily physical activity.
- One-third of American adults have high blood pressure.
- One in four American adults over age 60 has diabetes.

Many adults over age 50 wonder how the weight-creep and fitness decline happened. Susan and Tony are all too typical of what can happen as we age if food and fitness do not get enough attention over time. Susan rarely weighed herself and thought that a couple of extra pounds each year were no big deal as she aged. Adults of any age can relate to this feeling. Aging does have an effect on metabolism and hormones, making it easier to put on a few extra pounds. A few extra pounds are no big deal, but an extra 60 are a big deal. If Susan had monitored her weight, she might have given her weight creep some attention. Susan must have noticed that her dress size was going up each year, but she didn't halt the progress. Our health system doesn't help much either. How often do you get weighed at the doctor's office? Yet weight and exercise habits are frequently not addressed. Or maybe a discharge summary prints out a body mass index (BMI) score without any explanation of what it means. Studies show that when doctors talk to patients about their weight or about exercise, it helps promote behavior change, yet not enough doctors have a meaningful discussion with patients about how to change behavior when it comes to eating and exercise.

Tony is typical of the many former athletes we have worked with who thought they would always be active after being a high school or college athlete. Unless the person makes a conscious effort, fitness rapidly declines, muscle mass decreases, and body fat stores increase. While Tony's weight hasn't changed much, he has swapped lean muscle for fat, which is less dense but increases girth. As this book will point out, it doesn't take a superhuman effort to maintain fitness, and—more importantly for many—fitness can be regained at any age with a little commitment and effort. Throughout the book, you may see terms that may not be in your usual vocabulary, so flip to page 289 in the back of the book for some quick definitions.

Assess Yourself

In each chapter, you'll find a set of questions under the heading Assess Yourself that will help you evaluate your current habits. Take a few minutes to honestly answer the questions; don't worry, no one is grading your responses. As you read through the chapter, think about your answers to find out what you may be doing well and to learn what you could do to improve your food and fitness. Being honest with yourself is important because many people tend to overestimate their exercise effort and underestimate their food intake. For example, if an individual says that she plays tennis for an hour every day, how much of that time is spent in real activity? Is she playing doubles or rotating out for a set or two? Her hour of activity may be only 40 minutes long. Same with eating. You say you cook a healthy dinner every night, but in reality Friday night dinner is pizza night, and you usually order your pizza with sausage or pepperoni instead of healthier veggie options.

Let's assess your current habits by comparing them to your 25-year-old self. Think back and answer the questions in the Assess Yourself box on the next page and then read the review below.

ASSESS YOURSELF: IN REVIEW

How did you compare with your 25-year-old self? Are you happy and fit at your current weight, or would you like to gain or lose a few pounds? You'll learn more about healthy eating plans in Chapter 2, and if your goal is to lose or gain weight, Chapter 8 will provide more detailed advice. How about exercise habits? Are you meeting the minimum

Assess Yourself: The Basics

Compared with when I was 25, I weigh:

- ☐ more.
- ☐ less.
- ☐ the same.
- ☐ I don't know because I haven't weighed myself in a long time.

Compared with when I was 25, my eating habits have:

- ☐ improved.
- ☐ worsened.
- ☐ not changed.

When I was 25 it seemed that I could eat and drink whatever I wanted without gaining weight.

- ☐ True
- ☐ False

When I was 25 my job was:

- ☐ sedentary.
- ☐ mildly active.
- ☐ very active.

After age 25 my job(s) were mostly:

- ☐ sedentary.
- ☐ mildly active.
- ☐ very active.

At 25, my evenings were:

- ☐ sedentary.
- ☐ mildly active.
- ☐ very active.

Recently, my evenings have been mostly:

- ☐ sedentary.
- ☐ mildly active.
- ☐ very active.

I currently exercise less than when I was 25.

- ☐ True
- ☐ False

Exercise or physical activity was a normal part of my life when I was 25.

- ☐ True
- ☐ False

Exercise feels more challenging or difficult now than when I was 25.

- ☐ True
- ☐ False

I feel stiff and achy when I get out of a chair or off the couch compared with when I was 25.

- ☐ True
- ☐ False

Everyday conveniences (online banking, remote control for the television, cell phones, computers) have made me more sedentary than when I was 25.

- ☐ True
- ☐ False

I know my body composition (muscle versus fat) has changed since I was 25.

- ☐ Yes, for the better
- ☐ Yes, for the worse
- ☐ Unchanged
- ☐ Don't know

recommendations for exercise, including strength training? We will discuss exercise later in this chapter and in more detail in Section 2 (Move Well). You'll learn that increasing muscle mass can be the best way to boost metabolism (your body's rate of calorie burning) and increase strength and balance, all of which have many benefits. And, would you like to reduce the aches and pains of aging? Increasing flexibility (Chapter 7) can go a long way toward feeling and moving better every day. Use this initial assessment as a call to action to get motivated and make some changes that are outlined in the chapters that follow. Even though it may not be realistic to look and feel the same as you did at age 25, it is entirely possible to be healthy and fit as you age.

Clarifying the Science on Normal Aging

Age-Related Changes in Various Body Systems

As we age, every system in our body changes. Even though dozens of journals are devoted to the study of aging, researchers still find it hard to separate aging from disease. For example, is your difficulty opening a jar of olives the result of reduced grip strength (an aging effect) or arthritis (a disease effect)? It may be a bit of both, and throughout this book, we will offer strategies to help you deal with similar challenges. While aging cannot be stopped, the harmful effects of loss of muscle mass, poor balance, declining aerobic fitness, and the accumulation of excess body fat can be halted and even reversed with smart eating habits and the right physical activity. The phrase "use it or lose it" becomes true for many changes that are attributed to normal aging.

Let's take a brief look at the normal age changes in some of the body's systems. While none of us would say age 30 is old, that is about the age when changes in most of our body systems begin to occur. These changes occur gradually, and the good news is that aging adults can do many things to maintain good function, even at advanced ages. Also, bear in mind that these changes are highly individualized. Your father may have developed cataracts at age 60, while your 86-year-old mom may never develop cataracts severe enough to impair vision and require surgery. Another point to keep in mind is that while most aging adults experience decreased function compared with their 25-year-old selves, the body has tremendous reserve capacity. Thus, while the body may not be able to function at 100%, it can still function quite well in spite of modest declines. For example, you were born with two kidneys, but you can get by quite well with one—just ask a kidney donor!

Oxygen Uptake and Aerobic Capacity

Aging results in changes to aerobic fitness, which is measured by the ability to take in oxygen to power exercise. The best reflection of aerobic and cardiovascular fitness comes from a test called VO_2 max, shorthand for maximal oxygen consumption. Cycling or running to complete exhaustion is the typical way VO_2 max is measured. Around the age of 30, VO_2 max declines about 10% every decade in healthy adults, but older athletes see only about half that decline. Aging athletes who continue to perform endurance-type activities retain greater aerobic capacity than their couch-sitting friends of the same age. Aging will bring some decline to aerobic fitness, especially as you approach your 70s and 80s, but those who take up exercise in later life can expect to see their fitness level improve, even though they may never have the same fitness level as a 20-year-old athlete. Yet men and women over the age of 50 can and do partake in athletic competitions. Athletes competing in the National Senior Olympic Games experienced a 3.4% decrease in performance per year over 25 years of competition. This translates to a small decrease in performance from age 50 to 75, showing that regular participation in exercise can keep adults fit, and even competitive, into advanced age.

The decrease in VO_2 max is not fully understood, but experts believe the decrease comes from reduced training and a reduced maximal heart rate. Aging athletes may not have as much time to train at high levels as they did when they were younger; family and work responsibilities take time from training, and motivation may shift from setting personal best records to the health benefits of exercise. Yet the health benefits of exercise are a worthy goal for all adults over 50. We will show you how to improve your aerobic fitness in Chapter 5.

Body Composition

When we talk about body composition, we are referring to how much of your body is lean mass (muscle, organs, bone, skin) versus body fat. It is important to be mindful of the fact that body fat is essential for both men and women, so having zero body fat is not a healthy goal. However, aging seems to conspire to alter body composition; hormonal changes for women around menopause, specifically declining estrogen levels, along with declines in growth hormone levels, contribute to changes in body composition. With aging comes a tendency to see redistributed body fat, as more fat accumulates inside the abdomen (the dreaded belly fat) and less accumulates in the arms and legs. More information on managing body weight is found in Chapter 8.

Lack of physical activity is a major contributor to changes in body composition, but even aging athletes are not immune to weight gain or body composition changes. Exercise is one way to temper age-related weight gain. While the absolute amount of exercise needed to prevent weight gain is not known, one researcher tried to quantify physical activity with long-term weight change in over 34,000 American women who were not on any special diet. The women started the study when they were in their mid-50s, and researchers followed these women for 13 years. Weight and physical activity levels were measured at the start of the study and every 3 years throughout. At the end of the study, all women gained an average of 5 to 6 pounds. However, those who averaged 60 minutes a day of moderate-intensity exercise during the years of the study gained the least amount of weight, and the two less active groups of women were significantly more likely to gain more than 5 pounds. While some weight gain might be inevitable and acceptable, it is possible to prevent large weight gain with regular, moderate-intensity exercise.

Cardiovascular System

Regular physical exercise is the main pillar of prevention for cardiovascular disease. Aerobic exercise seems to confer benefits on lipid profiles compared with findings in sedentary older adults. Older athletes tend to have lipid profiles that reduce their risk for heart disease. The heart-protective effects of exercise may be in part due to the increase in high-density lipoprotein cholesterol (HDL-C) and the lowered ratio of total cholesterol to HDL-C. However, it appears that regular continuous exercise is needed to maintain a favorable lipid profile. If you were an athlete in high school, don't expect the benefits to cardiovascular health to still be there in your 60s if you haven't exercised in the intervening years.

Increases in body fat in the abdomen, insulin resistance, and high blood pressure are a cluster of conditions called metabolic syndrome, which increases risk for cardiovascular disease and type 2 diabetes. Exercise combined with healthy eating can help keep these conditions at bay.

Muscle Quantity and Quality

Age-related muscle loss usually begins at about age 40, when people lose about 10% to 15% in muscle mass and strength every 10 years. Progressive resistance strength training increases muscle mass and strength at every age. When it comes to muscle strength, it is never too late to begin a strength training program. A landmark study in the early 1990s showed that even among sedentary, older, nursing home residents (the oldest participant was 98 years old), muscle strength improved with regular resistance exercise. Enhanced muscle strength also improves walking gait and balance as people age. In reviewing many studies in older adults, one researcher found that strength training and increases in muscle mass in previously sedentary individuals resulted in a 1% increase in skeletal muscle size for each week of resistance training. While that may not turn an older adult into a superhero with rippling muscles, it can reverse decades of decline. Coupled with strength training is the need for more dietary protein as we age. Adults over age 50 need to eat more protein and should also distribute their intake evenly throughout the day. We'll discuss how much protein is needed and when to eat it for the best results in Chapter 6.

Blood Sugar Regulation

Aging brings about changes in how the body handles blood sugar (also called blood glucose), which comes from the digestion of carbohydrate in our diets. Fasting blood sugar levels tend to rise because our cells become more resistant to handling glucose as we age. It takes more insulin to move the glucose into cells. It is normal for blood sugar levels to rise and fall during a 24-hour period, depending on what and when we eat.

Two main hormones help keep blood sugar in a healthy range. One of those hormones is insulin, which is released by the pancreas after eating to help move blood sugar into muscles and other tissues for energy or storage. Between meals or overnight, when we are fasting, a hormone called glucagon is secreted to keep blood sugar levels in the normal range. Glucagon works by releasing sugar from storage in the liver. So, between the actions of these two hormones, blood sugar stays in a normal range, as illustrated below.

HOW THE PANCREAS RESPONDS TO LOW OR HIGH BLOOD GLUCOSE LEVELS

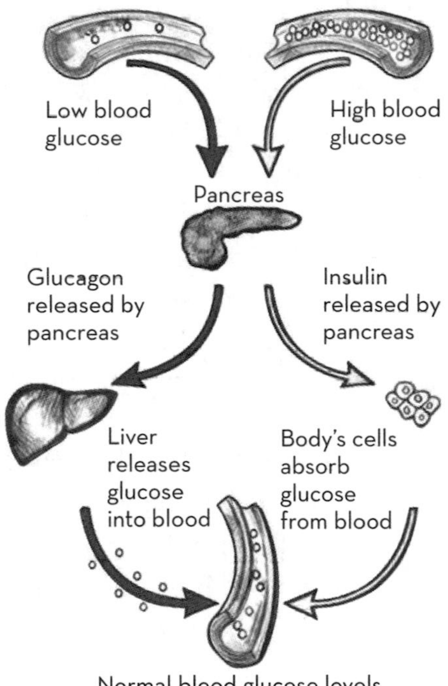

Reprinted from the National Institute of Diabetes and Digestive and Kidney Diseases, National Institutes of Health

Diabetes results when insulin is absent (type 1 diabetes) or cells become resistant to the action of insulin, and, therefore, insulin can't do its job as well as before (type 2 diabetes). Here is another instance where researchers believe that increased amounts of body fat coupled with chronic physical inactivity, rather than aging, is likely the real cause of insulin resistance. By measuring insulin resistance in various groups (younger and older endurance athletes, younger and older adults who were sedentary but remained at healthy weights, and younger and older adults who were obese), researchers showed that, regardless of age, the active groups were better able to use insulin and maintain normal blood sugar levels than either healthy weight or obese individuals. So, while it might be concluded that a higher blood sugar is a normal effect of aging, in fact, it is more likely associated with obesity and physical inactivity.

Gastrointestinal Tract

It's common to hear older adults complain about gut issues, but overall, the gastrointestinal tract functions well in the vast majority of healthy adults over age 50. The gastrointestinal tract includes all parts of the long tube that stretches from mouth to anus. Aging brings about slower movement of food and waste through the gastrointestinal tract, leading to a common complaint of constipation, which can be made worse by dehydration. Between 25% and 40% of older adults complain about constipation, yet simple dietary interventions can improve bowel health in most people. Interventions will be discussed in Chapters 2 and 3.

Gastric reflux, sometimes called heartburn because the pain is felt in the middle of the chest, affects about 20% of the population, and adults over age 50 are no more likely than younger adults to experience it. To reduce reflux, try implementing lifestyle interventions before taking over-the-counter meds, such as eating smaller meals, not eating late at night, and reducing fatty foods, all of which can help reduce reflux in most people.

Bones

Many people may not realize that bone is living tissue that is constantly undergoing change. Bone provides the framework that supports muscles, protects organs, and allows movement. It also is a vast reservoir of minerals like calcium, magnesium, and phosphorus. Up until about age 30, bone is constantly being remodeled; that is, new bone is made to replace older bone. But something happens around age 30 to slow that process, and it flips; less new bone is made, and more bone is lost—for both men and women. For women, the situation is even more pronounced: women have about 10% less bone mass overall compared to men, and women tend to get less bone-building nutrients in their diets, like calcium, protein, and magnesium. Then, around age 50, when menopause usually begins, the decrease in estrogen starts to further accelerate bone loss for women. However, both women and men can suffer from bone-thinning osteoporosis. Physical activity, coupled with increasing consumption of calcium, vitamin D, and protein, can help to minimize bone loss as we age. The impact of strength training on bone will be covered in Chapter 6.

Brain and Cognitive Function

Memory loss is a major concern for many aging adults. The minute their keys are misplaced or they leave an umbrella on the train, many people jump to the conclusion that they are one step away from dementia or Alzheimer's disease. If you have ever heard the words "senior moment" used when something is forgotten, you know what we mean. This is a term that we dislike. Both young and old forget from time to time. Aging does, however, bring about changes to the brain and how information is retrieved. Aging brains get smaller—especially the areas related to memory and learning complex tasks. Neurotransmitters, the chemical messengers that allow brain cells to talk to each other, may not work at maximum efficiency, and blood flow to the brain might change. However, like all other systems, the brain has reserve capacity. More importantly, the brain is "plastic," meaning it can grow and repair itself when it is regularly challenged.

Vision and Hearing Changes

It is no surprise that hearing and vision changes with age. The most common normal age change in vision occurs around age 40. *Presbyopia* is the term for the inability to read at close range; this manifests as needing to hold a book at arm's length to focus on the words. The solution is simple: bifocals, trifocals, or special contact lenses. Why is this important to food and fitness? Reading food labels is a useful tool in choosing healthy foods, so take reading glasses to the grocery store so you can investigate food labels and to restaurants so you can select healthier options. Sometimes vision is distorted, especially when a vision prescription changes, so be cautious when exercising, such as walking or jogging, over unfamiliar terrain. Your depth perception may be a bit off, which could lead to a fall.

Hearing losses occur later than vision changes; usually in the 60s. This condition, called *presbycusis*, is the gradual loss of hearing as we age. Some adults have hearing loss from exposure to loud noises from their occupation: musicians, lawn care workers, and some in the military experience hearing loss. There is concern that younger generations will have more severe hearing loss, and will have it earlier, due to the ubiquitous ear buds that are used to listen to music. Hearing loss can impair social relationships and make it hard to respond to warnings. Nobody wants to admit they have hearing loss, but it negatively affects quality of life, so talking to your doctor about solutions is a necessary, but perhaps unpleasant, fact of aging.

Hair, Skin, and Nail Changes

The integumentary system encompasses the hair, skin, and nails, all of which are designed to be physical barriers protecting the body from the outside world. This body system will most likely show the first visual signs of aging. The amount, color, and texture of hair, for example, changes as we age, but as with every body system, the changes are highly individualized. The growth and structure of nails also changes as we get older, although it is hard to determine how much change is true aging and how much is due to environmental exposure. Nails that are frequently soaked in water in occupations such as dishwashing, pet grooming, or hairdressing are more likely to be weak and soft. Women who use artificial nails or heavy coats of nail polish may find their nails more damaged as they age. The skin loses elasticity and resilience as we age, resulting in fine lines, wrinkles, and laxness. Skin layers become thin, especially on the hands. A lifetime of exposure to the sun's rays can also take a toll on the skin: rough texture, leathery appearance, and age spots are more noticeable with chronic sun exposure. In the United States, millions are spent on skin, hair, and nail products that promise dramatic reversal of the visual effects of aging, but according to the American Dermatological Association, simple solutions like protecting the skin from the sun, using moisturizer, exercising, getting enough sleep, and eating healthy are more likely to be beneficial than "miracle" age-erasing creams and lotions.

Benefits of Exercise and Healthy Eating in Adults

Exercise

We use the word exercise reluctantly because, for many people, exercise conjures up demotivating images of uncomfortable drudgery. Throughout this book, we'll use different synonyms for exercise, such as physical activity, working out, and training, in the hope that readers will relate to at least one of those terms in a positive way. Regardless of what we call it, the benefits of exercise are well known, and most people say they feel better when they are physically active on a regular basis. As you begin to evaluate your current exercise habits, consider these guidelines for physical activity from the US Office of Disease Prevention and Health Promotion:

- Set a goal for yourself of 2 hours and 30 minutes (150 minutes) of moderate-intensity aerobic activity every week (or 75 minutes of vigorous-intensity aerobic activity) and engage in muscle-strengthening exercise that works all major muscle groups on two or more days a week.
- For even greater benefits, strive to engage in 5 hours (300 minutes) of moderate-intensity activity or 2 hours and 30 minutes (150 minutes) of vigorous activity (or a combination of these activities) every week.
- The guidelines point out that when older adults cannot meet these recommendations, they should be as physically active as their abilities and conditions will allow. Exercises that maintain or improve balance are especially important to reduce the risk of falling.

We'll be referring to these guidelines throughout the book and discussing them in more detail in Section 2 (Move Well) because they represent a minimum goal that people of all ages should strive to achieve. Remember, only one in five adults meets these minimum physical activity guidelines. Consider the many benefits of regular exercise:

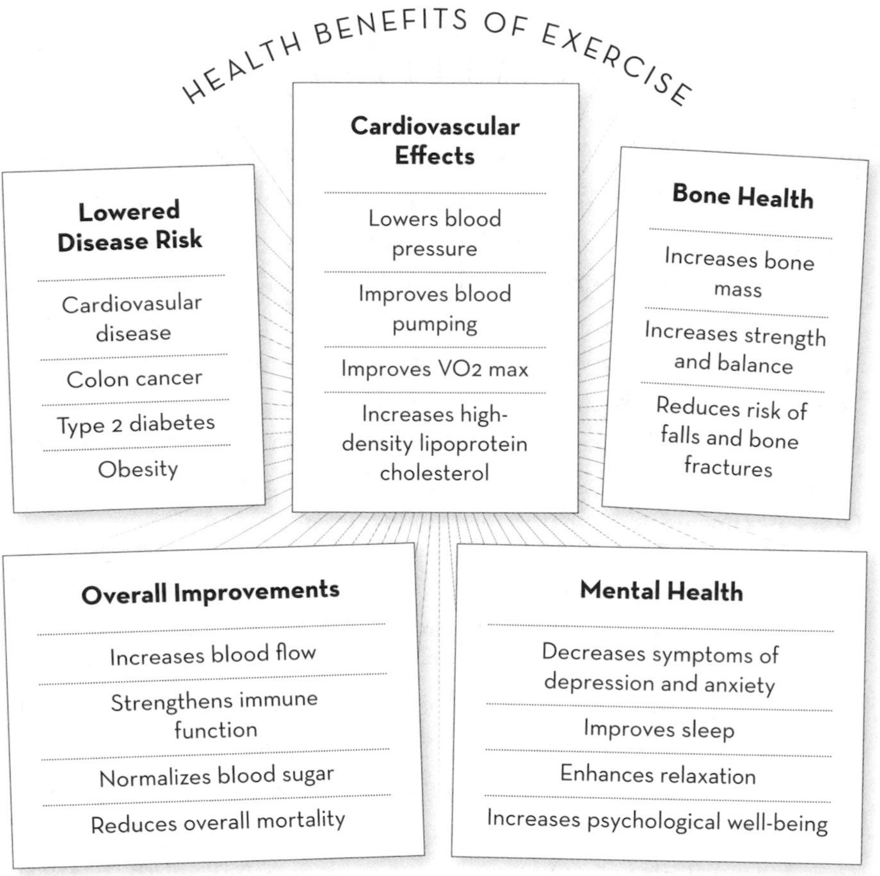

In addition to the individual physical and psychological benefits, exercise has significant societal benefits. Healthy, active older adults typically have reduced health care costs and enhanced productivity, thereby promoting a positive and active image of aging adults for younger generations to emulate.

Healthy Eating

Hunger and thirst are basic physical needs. But, who hasn't eaten when he or she wasn't hungry and drank when not thirsty, even knowing that these behaviors can be counterproductive for health goals and weight control. We want you to enjoy the foods you like but learn to evaluate food choices and portion sizes to help you become healthier.

Everyone wants to know which are the best foods to eat and information on superfoods that can cure all ills. Sorry to disappoint so soon in the book, but there is no one food that will meet all your nutritional needs, support healthy aging, prevent disease, and make skin glow. Individual nutrients are important for good health, but people rarely eat single nutrients; they eat foods that contain a variety of nutrients in a total package that may have synergistic (com-

Dietary Approaches to Stop Hypertension (DASH) Plan

DASH is based on an eating pattern developed to lower blood pressure. The plan is rich in fruits, vegetables, low-fat dairy foods, pulses (beans and peas), seafood, poultry, whole grains, and nuts. These foods contain the minerals potassium, calcium, and magnesium, which seem to help lower blood pressure.

Flexitarian Eating Plan

A flexitarian eat plan is a plant-based eating pattern that is mostly vegetarian but allows for the flexibility of eating animal protein on occasion.

Mediterranean Diet

The Mediterranean diet eating pattern is based on the diets of people who live in countries surrounding the Mediterranean Sea. The plan is rich in olive oil, nuts, pulses (beans and peas), vegetables, fruit, fish, poultry, and whole grains.

Mediterranean-DASH Intervention for Neurodegenerative Delay (MIND) Diet

As the name implies, this eating pattern combines the DASH and Mediterranean diets. The eating pattern focuses on leafy green vegetables, nuts, berries, whole grains, fish, poultry, and olive oil.

plementary) effects when consumed together. While there are no true superfoods, there are super diets. We want to focus on healthy eating patterns as the best approach to optimal aging. The other reason we like the concept of healthy eating patterns is that people don't eat one diet to strengthen bones, another for heart health, and a different one for weight loss. We encourage an eating plan to support all health goals. Several healthy eating plans will be introduced in Chapter 2 that can be customized to work for anyone. The plans, along with brief definitions, are described on the previous page.

Confronting Myths About Aging

Some people think aging is out of their control; the truth is that adults over age 50 can do many things to stay healthy as they age, and they can essentially turn back the clock in terms of how their bodies function. Instead of throwing up our hands and using fallback excuses, let's take a look at common beliefs about aging and set the record straight.

MYTH: Genetics is more important than lifestyle when it comes to controlling disease.

REALITY: There's no doubt genetics plays a role in many things in our lives. Eye color, hair texture, dimples, or a cleft chin are all due to genes; diet and physical activity won't do anything to change them. For many, the genes we inherited for conditions such as obesity or heart disease can interact with our lifestyle choices and behaviors to produce excess body fat or blocked arteries. In other words, genetics *and* lifestyle are important determinants of our health. So, while we may have inherited a stocky body type or a higher risk for heart disease, obesity or coronary bypass surgery isn't the inevitable result. A recent study on genetic risk, adherence to a healthy lifestyle, and coronary disease found a 46% lower risk of disease in those who had healthy lifestyles, despite the fact that they were at a high genetic risk for heart disease. Lifestyle factors, such as diet, exercise, and maintaining a healthy weight, are also tied to the most common cancers. In fact, the American Institute for Cancer Research estimates that about one-third of cancer cases are preventable through changes in lifestyle.

MYTH: It takes too much time to get fit or eat right.

REALITY: We all have the same 1,440 minutes in a day, but how we choose to use them is under our control. We find time to binge-watch our favorite television shows, click away at internet stories, or surf Facebook for hours at a time. Yet, we can also use some of those minutes to plan our meals for the week so that we have a fridge and pantry stocked with healthy foods or so that we can schedule time for being more active. Give some serious thought to where activity can fit into your day, every day. Sign up for group exercise classes (do you get free or reduced gym membership fees with your supplemental Medicare insurance?), get a dog, or visit the local animal shelter and walk a dog every day.

MYTH: It is too hard to cook for one or two people.

REALITY: It might be different from cooking for a family, but cooking for yourself or for you and someone else is not difficult. You can scale back recipes, or you can continue to cook for a crowd but freeze portions so you can cook once and eat multiple times.

MYTH: It takes a gym membership to get fit.

REALITY: You can get fit without signing up for expensive gym memberships, hiring personal trainers, or buying exercise equipment. Chapters 5, 6, and 7 are devoted to simple ways to get and stay fit without joining a gym.

MYTH: It is only a matter of time before all older people get dementia.

REALITY: While we hear about the seemingly growing numbers of older adults with Alzheimer's disease, it is important to remember that this is a disease, not a normal part of aging. Researchers are finding that modifying our behavior can help preserve brain function. Emerging research suggests that the following can help keep our brains sharp:

- Regular social interactions
- Consistent physical activity
- Maintaining a sense of purpose
- Remaining conscientious
- Keeping a healthy cardiovascular system, including controlling blood pressure
- Eating fruits and vegetables
- Engaging in learning activities that involve memory, reasoning, and processing speed

Commonly Asked Questions About Aging

Is it necessary to watch my diet if I am taking a statin or blood pressure or diabetes medications to control my disease?

Medications are not a replacement for lifestyle interventions. The small-type, printed inserts that come with prescription meds indicate that the drugs work best when paired with a healthy diet. For those who take statins to lower cholesterol, it is wise to regularly choose heart-healthy foods. There is no question that a grilled salmon salad beats a bacon cheeseburger for heart health, even if you do take a statin. Blood pressure drugs work best in concert with lower-sodium diets, and blood-sugar–lowering drugs work best with a diet higher in fiber and lower in simple sugars. An added benefit of healthy food choices is that many times drugs can be eliminated or the dosage reduced—changes that are good for your health and your wallet.

Is it more expensive to eat healthy foods?

Eating right doesn't have to be expensive. There are many ways to eat better without breaking the bank. The easiest way to save money on groceries is to plan ahead; plan meals, know what foods or ingredients are needed to prepare these meals, make a list, and go shopping. The people who say it takes too much time to plan are the same folks who run to the grocery store two or three times a week or stop at the drive-through window. Sticking to a plan also helps curb unnecessary impulse buying. Consider trying private-label brands and switching to the ones that are acceptable substitutes. Buy in season when you can; for example, strawberries are less expensive in the summer and often cost more in the winter. Consider joining a community-supported agriculture (CSA) plan from a local farmer. You will not only get fresh produce but also learn how to efficiently use your new veggies so as not to waste the produce. Roasted turnips or kale smoothies might just surprise you!

Having the Confidence to Make Food and Fitness Work for You

As we move through the next several chapters, we will help you find food and fitness plans that work for your lifestyle. We understand that one size does not fit all. Some people love to work out in a home gym, some can't wait until their next group exercise class at the gym, and others are happy to walk in their neighborhood. Our goal is to help you recognize that improving your health need not be daunting. Everyone can take small steps each day toward better health. And doing so doesn't have to be difficult or self-defeating. There's no need to feel guilty when you don't reach a daily fitness goal or after you eat a meal that is higher in calories. We want to encourage you to continue to set realistic goals, but not to beat yourself up if you don't achieve them. We want you to enjoy your favorite foods and balance what you eat throughout the day to fuel your physical activity and give you the energy you need to accomplish your goals.

Remember Susan and Tony from the opening paragraphs of this chapter? Susan experienced weight creep by not monitoring her weight as the years went by. It behooves all of us, at any age, to monitor our health, including our weight. Prevention is a better strategy than treatment. But it isn't too late for Susan; after self-reflection, Susan joined a local YMCA and, together with her husband, made a commitment to work out an hour each day. Added to that commitment was the decision to subscribe to a healthy home meal-delivery kit. Susan and her husband prepare meals together, eat a healthier diet, and enjoy the time spent together. Susan knows she may never be the same weight she was at 25, but she also knows she can be healthy and fit as she ages.

Tony realized that he still has the will and discipline he had when he was a young athlete and decided to channel that desire into improving his health. His doctor explained that prediabetes is a warning and that changing his lifestyle could prevent him from developing full-blown diabetes. Tony started increasing his fitness by doing little things, such as walking every morning before work, walking the dog after work, climbing the three flights of stairs to his office instead of taking the elevator, and packing a healthy lunch instead of eating out every day. He purchased a home blood glucose test kit and found that his blood sugar level was decreasing as he increased his activity and improved his diet. Motivated by his small steps, Tony joined a group to start training for a 5K road race.

We hope that, like Susan and Tony, you will find a few things you are willing to focus on to be healthier and more fit. It doesn't take much to get on the path to better health, and the following chapters will lay out strategies, tips, and ideas to help you on your journey. Many healthy adults have successfully adopted the lifestyle changes discussed in this book as they've aged and are still following them. You can do it, too!

Conversation with an Expert

Julie Miller Jones, PhD, LN, CNS, professor emerita at St Catherine University in St Paul, MN, has seen a lot of changes in the nutrition world in her 70 years. She knows nutrition and exercise have played a big part in her professional success and her active lifestyle. "I am one of the few who eat according to the *2015–2020 Dietary Guidelines for Americans*," she says. It is estimated that only 3% to 8% of Americans follow the dietary advice found in the guidelines. Julie eats not only for good nutrition but also for taste, explaining: "I have been a James Beard Award [cookbook] judge, so cooking and taste is paramount. I think great taste makes adhering to the *Dietary Guidelines* easier."

Julie works tirelessly to set the record straight on grains in an effort to help people understand that they're not evil:

> My husband and I are big proponents of eating whole grains and fibers and miss them if we are on the road and cannot get them. At home during the week, my breakfast usually consists of oatmeal with some oat bran and other multigrain cereal that I make on Monday to enjoy for the rest of the week. When traveling and dining out, I love it when the bread choice has whole grains. With all the focus on gut health and the microbiome, we also now think about the importance of fiber and its role in health and a healthy gut.

Julie and her husband are adventurous cooks:

> I use cooking magazines and my cookbook collection to plan meals. My husband usually shops or, in season, we enjoy going to the farmers' markets together. We often cook together. Dinners rarely ever include the same dish because there are so many foods in the world to taste and so little time. So we cook from all cultures and with unusual ingredients. My husband is a wine aficionado, and so we enjoy it with our dinners and our restaurant outings.

Physical activity is also part of the *Dietary Guidelines* advice. Julie does yoga every day when she is home. "I *adore* yoga," she says, "especially in a class which forces me to work harder than I would on my own." When traveling, Julie walks the city she is visiting or does some biking and water aerobics. Julie's philosophy is simple: "Food and health are such a beautiful piece of life. Take time to foster them and enjoy them. Healthy food can be fun, delicious, and part of the adventure of life. And it helps you to feel well enough to enjoy it all."

Useful Resources

Centers for Disease Control and Prevention (www.cdc.gov/aging/aginginfo/index.htm)

- ▷ *Health information for older adults, including physical activity and nutrition among many other topics*

Healthy Aging (https://healthyaging.net)

- ▷ *Information on food, lifestyle, and exercise*

Mayo Clinic (www.mayoclinic.org/healthy-lifestyle/healthy-aging/in-depth/aging/art-20046070)

- ▷ *What to expect as we age and what to do about it*

National Institute on Aging (www.nia.nih.gov/health)

- ▷ *Addresses a variety of health and aging topics*

National Institute of Diabetes and Digestive and Kidney Diseases (www.niddk.nih.gov/health-information)

- ▷ *Information on diabetes; diseases of the digestive tract, the kidney, the liver, the urinary tract, and the endocrine systems; and weight management, diet, and nutrition*

The Office of Disease Prevention and Health Promotion (https://health.gov)

- ▷ *Covers the Physical Activity Guidelines for Americans and the latest Dietary Guidelines for Americans*

SECTION 1

EAT WELL

IN THIS SECTION of the book, we take a deep dive into what eating well means. Although the title of the section is Eat Well, we also include a chapter devoted to hydration. Most of you can probably name the nutrients—carbohydrate, protein, fat, vitamins, and minerals—but many overlook the sixth essential and crucial nutrient, water.

The phrase "you are what you eat" is thought to be attributed to a French physician in the 1820s who said, "Tell me what you eat, and I will tell you what you are." In our modern world of fast and processed food, that could be translated into "If you are what you eat, are you fast, cheap, and easy?"

Eating well is a habit that most adults recognize as being important. We all know firsthand that we can't eat and drink the same way we did when we were younger if we want to maintain our body weight and keep blood sugar, blood lipid, and blood pressure levels in check. A 2016 survey from the International Food Information

Council Foundation on food and health found that those aged 52 to 70 years old were more likely than other generations to consider health when deciding on food purchases. But the challenge in determining what constitutes healthy is that we are bombarded with nutrition advice from celebrities, television doctors, media headlines, and well-meaning friends and family. From website headings touting the "five superfoods you should eat today" to social media posts that scare us into believing our food supply is toxic, it is no wonder that adults of all ages are confused about foods.

We encourage you to stop searching for the elixir of youth through food, drink, or dietary supplements and to adopt a healthy eating plan for life. The *2015–2020 Dietary Guidelines for Americans* emphasizes eating patterns, not a prescribed intake of carbohydrate, protein, or fat. Several position papers from the Academy of Nutrition and Dietetics also herald dietary patterns for good health. There is no doubt that diet can improve blood lipids, glucose and insulin levels, blood pressure, and body fat; abnormal values for all of these are major risk factors for chronic diseases. Yet fewer than 1% of adults follow a diet that meets the American Heart Association 2020 goals. In this section, we present four different eating plans and show you how they might fit your lifestyle. We encourage you to eat more of the good stuff at every meal (whole grains; fruits; vegetables; legumes, such as beans, peas, and lentils; lean meat; fish; seafood; dairy foods; nuts; and vegetable oils) and eat less of the rest. Remember: eat less doesn't mean eat never. Food is something that should be enjoyed, but we should flip our thinking that eating well means deprivation or a Spartan diet of cleanses and juicing. Food can be nutritious and delicious, and it should be both, not one or the other.

This section also provides real-food examples of how to get the micronutrients and nutrients—including vitamins, minerals, and important plant compounds, called phytonutrients—that are needed in small amounts in your diet yet are so important to good health. Food is the best matrix for delivering nutrients. While we recommend getting nutrients from foods, there are times when supplementation makes sense, and we encourage you to use the information on dietary supplements to be informed about what you are taking and why you are taking a supplement.

We encourage you to assess your food-related habits and beliefs at the beginning of each chapter and use your responses to guide your decisions about improving your food choices and hydration practices and create an eating plan for good health and good taste.

Aging is not an excuse to eat and drink whatever and whenever you want or to spend your days being sedentary, as that will only hasten the aging process. But aging doesn't start when we are 50 years old; most of our body systems start to show some decline in our 30s and 40s. The term *plasticity* is often used to describe the ability of body tissues and organs to respond to a stimulus, such as better eating (and activity) habits, to improve function. Don't assume that blood sugar, blood lipids, blood pressure, and body fat will rise to unhealthy levels as a normal part of aging. All can be kept in check with healthy eating and physical activity, no matter your age.

CHAPTER

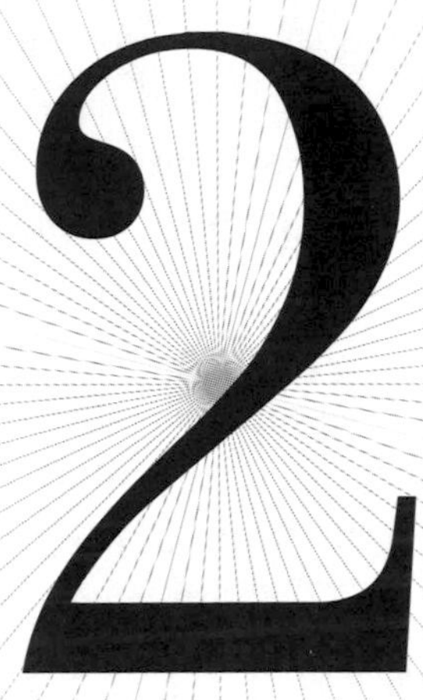

EATING FOR OPTIMAL AGING

The Bottom Line

Many healthy eating plans promote optimal aging, but when it comes to choosing the right plan, it can be hard to sort through conflicting information about which diet is best and which food currently claims the title of superfood. Celebrities, talk show doctors, personal trainers, magazine and online headlines, and your friends are all whispering in your ear, telling you what to eat or not to eat. It is as if everyone who eats is a nutrition expert, and they all have an opinion about what you should be putting on your plate. Instead of telling you what is best, we offer four different eating plans backed by science that contain a variety of healthy foods from all food groups that, best of all, taste great. The plans (introduced in Chapter 1) are the Dietary Approaches to Stop Hypertension (DASH) eating plan, the Flexitarian eating plan, a Mediterranean-style eating plan, and the Mediterranean-DASH Intervention for Neurodegenerative Delay (MIND) eating plan.

Keep these key points in mind as you consider changing your eating pattern:

- **There is no best diet or best food. There are many healthy eating plans, and there is bound to be one plan that works best for you.**
- **A healthy eating plan should contain a balance of the three major nutrients (also known as macronutrients)—carbohydrates, proteins, and fats. We don't advocate for a high-this and low-that diet. Instead, we want you to focus on eating enough fruits, vegetables, whole grains, nuts, seeds, protein-rich foods, and healthy fats and oils.**
- **An optimal-aging diet contains nutrient-rich foods that provide the nutrients needed for healthy aging without overdoing calories.**
- **Even small changes in your diet can make a difference to your health. Start small and work your way to a healthy way of eating every day. Enjoy all foods in moderation, make healthy choices when you can, and learn to make substitutions, not sacrifices.**
- **Cooking is the best way to make healthy meals. Highly processed packaged and frozen foods are often high in sodium, sugar, and less-healthy fats.**

Introduction

Everyone wants to know what is *best*—the best food, the best diet, the best exercise—for optimal aging. Here's a not-so-secret secret: there is no best. We are going to show you that black-and-white thinking about what is "best" generally leads to frustration and disappointment. We get frustrated because one day we may hear that a low-carb, high-fat diet is best, and then someone else comes along another day and says a vegan diet, high in carbs and low in fat, is best. Disappointment is inevitable for those who go on and off the latest diets, always seeking the best. As much as everyone complains that food and nutrition advice is ever-changing, consider the following:

- Nutrition is a science, not an art, and science evolves. A sensible eating plan, though, takes into account both art and science—art because it can be personalized and designed for you, and science because it follows available research. Nothing in science is revolutionary; it is evolutionary. Forty years ago, scientists had good reason to believe cholesterol in foods contributed to high blood cholesterol. Now we know that dietary cholesterol has less of an effect on blood cholesterol than other types of fats, like *trans* fats and some saturated fats, as well as excess refined carbohydrates (carbs).

- Food and nutrition headlines are meant to grab your attention and get you to click on an article, turn the page, or stay tuned to hear the story. Too often, the headline doesn't match the story content. Consider this recent headline, "Study shows red wine can help burn body fat, prevent obesity." That headline made us want to break out the pinot noir! But hold on for the full story. The researchers found that when female mice were fed a compound called resveratrol (found in red grapes) along with a special diet, the color of their fat changed. Although this change in fat color has been *linked* to burning more calories, keep in mind that "linked" doesn't mean the same thing as "caused," and research in mice shouldn't be the basis for changing food choices.
- It's tempting to believe in magic. Who among us doesn't want to believe that a simple solution is the answer to a complex problem? Even though science can't back up the claims that raspberry ketones or green tea extract will melt away the pounds, if these products (or products like them) are touted as miracle supplements on a popular television show, they often sell like hotcakes, practically overnight. If it sounds too good to be true, it's very likely that it is, and the magic you anticipate is unlikely to happen.
- When adopting an eating plan that severely limits a food group, we often find that the substitutions that are made may have unintended consequences. For example, when low-fat diets were all the rage, food manufacturers replaced fat with sugar. Most of us remember the low-fat cookie craze of the 1990s. And when we give up dairy milk for healthy-sounding almond

milk, we also lose the protein found in dairy milk—8 g of protein in 1 cup of cow's milk versus 1 g in almond milk. Dairy milk also provides more potassium, magnesium, calcium, and phosphorus than almond milk.

So where does that leave us? The fact is that no one food or diet is best. There are many good foods and eating plans, and this chapter will present four dietary patterns that support optimal aging.

Here are some of the key principles that make up an optimal diet for the 50+ population:

- *Inclusion of all energy-containing nutrients (energy refers to calories)*

  Carbohydrate, protein, and fat are included in every plan featured here. These diets might contain different mixes of these macronutrients, but they are not high-protein, low-fat or low-carb diets. Instead, these diets feature a healthy balance of all nutrients.

- *A focus on nutrient-rich foods*

  Many older adults need fewer calories as they age unless they are very physically active. To maintain a healthy body weight, most of us need to be more selective in our food choices. There is less room in your diet for a pitcher of beer and a basket of fried chicken wings, than there was when you were younger. Although these foods are not off-limits, smaller portions can still be enjoyed. Instead, focus on foods that are nutritious, delicious, and filling.

- *Concern for disease risk*

  We chose eating plans that reduce the risk of the most common chronic diseases of aging: heart disease, high blood pressure, diabetes, osteoporosis, and arthritis. Foods that are good sources of nutrients and compounds that reduce inflammation are hallmarks of the eating plans in this chapter.

- *Enjoyment of eating and mealtime*

  Food is so much more than the sum of its nutrients; food is an essential and enjoyable part of life. Share meals with family and friends. Experiment with new flavors and new recipes. Eat for health most of the time, but recognize that everything in moderation is just fine. Of course, the problem is that many of us don't know what moderation really means. Sharing a decadent dessert with your dinner companions is moderation; ordering the death-by-chocolate cake for yourself is not.

ASSESS YOURSELF: IN REVIEW

Before moving on, take the Assess Yourself quiz on the next page. Then, keep reading.

The goal of this assessment is to make you more aware of your habits and beliefs about food and eating. Among the many healthy eating patterns and information presented in this chapter, we will introduce four eating styles, one or more of which might work for you. Regardless of your current eating plan and habits, some basic advice holds true: try to eat regular meals, spaced throughout the day, without back-loading your calories at night. Eat regular meals with plenty of fiber and protein to help satisfy and reduce hunger. Consider your portion sizes (for more on portion sizes and weight control, see Chapter 8) because you can overeat healthy foods, too. Also, consider your health goals and determine if your current eating style is supporting them, whether your goal is to reduce your risk for chronic disease, manage an existing condition, lower your high blood pressure, or keep your blood lipid values in check. The good news about all of these eating plans is that they can hit many targets: controlling chronic diseases, reducing inflammation, managing weight, and supporting exercise.

Assess Yourself: Current Eating Habits

What do you usually eat for breakfast? (Let's define breakfast as what you eat—beyond a cup of coffee—within 1 hour after getting out of bed.)

How many times a day do you eat?

- ☐ Less than three
- ☐ Three or four
- ☐ More than four

How are your meals usually spaced throughout the day? How many hours between eating occasions?

- ☐ 3 to 4 hours
- ☐ 5 to 6 hours
- ☐ 7 or more hours

What is the size of each meal and snack? For example, do you eat a light breakfast and lunch, an afternoon snack, and then a big evening meal? Rate each eating occasion as small, medium, or large in terms of the number of calories you think you typically consume.

Breakfast

- ☐ Small (<400 calories)
- ☐ Medium (400 to 500 calories)
- ☐ Large (>500 calories)

Lunch

- ☐ Small (<400 calories)
- ☐ Medium (400 to 500 calories)
- ☐ Large (>500 calories)

Dinner

- ☐ Small (<400 calories)
- ☐ Medium (400 to 500 calories)
- ☐ Large (>500 calories)

Do the foods you eat make you feel:

- ☐ satisfied?
- ☐ hungry sooner after eating than you'd like?

What protein-rich foods/drinks do you consume and when?

Do you avoid carbohydrates?

- ☐ Yes
- ☐ No

  If yes, do you:

  - ☐ avoid all carbs?
  - ☐ just certain types of carbs?

What type of fat do you use for cooking, as a spread, or in salad dressings?

- ☐ Mostly saturated fats
- ☐ Mostly unsaturated fats

What foods/drinks do you try to avoid (or minimize) and why?

Do you have any specific goals that influence what you eat? Choose all that apply.

- ☐ I'd like to lose weight.
- ☐ I'd like to maintain my current weight.
- ☐ I'd like to alter my body composition to improve muscle tone and strength.
- ☐ I'd like to gain weight, especially muscle.
- ☐ I want to eat foods that curb my appetite.
- ☐ I want to eat foods that give me more energy.
- ☐ I try to avoid foods and drinks that cause reflux or bloating.
- ☐ I just enjoy eating and usually don't associate it with health outcomes.
- ☐ I need to eat foods that help keep my cholesterol under control.
- ☐ I need to eat foods that keep my blood pressure under control.
- ☐ I need to eat certain foods to manage my diabetes.
- ☐ I have other medical concerns that influence what I eat.

Choose Your Healthy Eating Plan

We will present four healthy eating plans that we believe work well for most adults over age 50. For each plan described in the chart on the next page, recommended carbohydrate-, protein-, and fat-containing foods are provided, as well as foods to eat less of. It is easy to see that all four eating plans have many things in common: eat more fruits, vegetables, whole grains, and healthy fats and oils; eat less sugar-containing foods, saturated fats, and sodium. Many people will be glad to know that all four plans also include alcohol in moderation. The Mediterranean diet suggests red wine for those who drink alcohol, but the other plans don't specify alcohol type. Our suggestion on alcohol is this: if you drink alcohol, moderate your intake to one or two drinks a day for men and one drink a day for women. Remember, not drinking during the week and drinking it all on Saturday night is not moderation; that is binge drinking. If you don't drink alcohol, don't start because you think it might be healthy. The dangers of excess alcohol are real. Alcohol also contains calories, and more than one or two drinks can impact your ability to stick to a healthy eating plan. So if you enjoy beer, wine, or cocktails, do so in moderation. More information on alcohol intake with an illustration of what is considered a single drink is found in Chapter 8.

Mediterranean Diet

David, a 66-year-old cyclist, eats one meal a day—dinner—to control his weight. David cycles about 75 miles each week and takes part in many regional cycling events, including century (100-mile) bike rides. Lately, he has complained of being tired during his long rides, and he believes he is losing muscle mass. He eats plenty of simple carbs during his long rides, mostly gels and sports drinks, but he wonders if his one-meal-a-day plan is sabotaging his workouts as he is getting older. David loves to cook and enjoys trying new dishes, but he is stuck on the one-good-meal-a-day plan. David's fatigue and loss of muscle are telling him that he is not fueling his body to support his exercise. Maintaining and

EATING PLAN	Recommended Carbohydrate Foods	Recommended Protein Foods	Recommended Fats	Eat Less of These Foods
Mediterranean	Fruits, vegetables, whole grains	Mostly fish and other seafood, and beans (legumes), with eggs, cheese, poultry, and yogurt in moderation	Olive oil, nuts	Red meat, processed meat, sweets, sugar-sweetened beverages
Dietary Approaches to Stop Hypertension (DASH)	Fruits, vegetables, whole grains	Low-fat dairy, lean meat, poultry, fish, beans	Vegetable oils, nuts	Sweets, sugar-sweetened beverages, tropical oils (coconut, palm, or palm kernel), salty foods
Flexitarian	Fruits, vegetables, whole grains	Tofu, lentils, peas, nuts, seeds, and beans and occasional seafood, poultry, or meat	Vegetable and olive oils	Meat and animal foods, sweets
Mediterranean-DASH Intervention for Neuro-degenerative Delay (MIND)	Whole grains, berries, green leafy vegetables	Fish, poultry, beans, nuts	Not specified	Red meat, butter, stick margarine, sweets, pastries, full-fat cheese, fried foods, fast foods

building muscle requires a moderate increase in dietary protein and distribution of protein throughout the day. His one meal a day may help him control his calorie intake, but it is sabotaging his fitness goals.

Over 45 years ago, a Minnesota researcher named Ancel Keys published a study on the dietary patterns of people who live in countries that surround the Mediterranean Sea. He wanted to know how dietary patterns affect the risk of developing heart disease. Keys reported that the people in this region who ate the local, traditional diet rich in olive oil, whole grains, beans, fruits, and vegetables and who ate fish and meat in moderation had a significantly decreased rate of heart disease deaths than people who ate other diets. This regional dietary pattern came to be known as the Mediterranean diet. Over time, many more studies have shown that adhering to a Mediterranean diet lowers the risk of coronary heart disease, heart attack, and stroke.

Let's be clear about a Mediterranean diet: there isn't just one eating plan. It can be based on the dietary patterns of any particular country that borders the Mediterranean Sea, such as Greece, Italy, or Spain. No matter the country, all have core foods and nutrients that are included. The foods in the plan are rich in the healthy fats found in olive oil and nuts and contain plant-based proteins, like legumes, along with fish (the countries are located by a sea, after all), poultry, and whole grains. Mediterranean foods are also high in antioxidant nutrients, like vitamins A, C, and E, as well as the mineral selenium. Subsequent research has also identified that many of the foods included in this style of eating also have anti-inflammatory properties.

Let's also be clear about what a Mediterranean diet is not. When Americans adopt a country's cuisine, they tend to change it to meet American tastes—and not necessarily for the better. Pouring olive oil over all-you-can-eat breadsticks or drowning pasta in Alfredo sauce and adding Italian sausage is not a healthy version of the Mediterranean diet. A true Mediterranean diet is simple food, simply prepared, using herbs and spices for flavor. However, we are not trying to be the food police; we believe all foods can fit, but they can't fit all of the time. If you love Alfredo sauce, you don't have to give it up forever.

Make marinara the default sauce for your pasta, and save Alfredo sauce as the occasional topping.

Why It Might Work for You

A Mediterranean eating plan works for many people: those who want to reduce their risk of heart disease or high blood pressure, as well as those who are healthy and simply enjoy good food. We think this plan would work for David, the cyclist. By eating one meal a day, David doesn't have enough energy to get through long bike rides. Distributing protein-rich foods throughout the day helps create a muscle-building environment, instead of a muscle-losing one (learn more about this in Chapter 6). David likes to cook, and the Mediterranean-style diet offers a variety of healthy foods. He can experiment with flavors from Italy, Spain, Greece, and northern African countries. Below is a sample meal plan that will help David stay fueled without feeling too full on days when he has long rides.

Breakfast	Greek yogurt with chopped nuts and dried fruit, coffee, a fresh peach, and tart cherry juice or pomegranate juice
Lunch	Mediterranean chopped salad topped with feta cheese and albacore tuna, whole grain crackers, marinated olives, and sparkling water with lemon
Dinner	Grilled cod with roasted cherry tomatoes and other vegetables, whole wheat pita bread, and a glass of red wine or red grape juice
Snacks	Dried fruit-and-nut mix to be eaten during long bike rides, fresh fruit and vegetables with hummus, and plenty of water. Include sports drinks on hot, humid days during long rides.

Dietary Approaches to Stop Hypertension (DASH)

Caroline has read many diet books, and she has concluded that a low-carb diet is the best approach for her. At age 56, she has explored every low-carb diet from the Atkins diet to the Wheat Belly diet. She loses about 5 pounds within the first few days of the diet and feels great, but after a couple of weeks, her weight loss slows, and she goes off the diet, only to see the pounds come back on. Caroline is, by her estimation, 15 pounds overweight, and she is tired of the cycle of weight loss and weight regain. A recent diagnosis of mild hypertension makes her wonder: what is the best approach to manage both her weight and her high blood pressure? Carolyn is chasing popular diets only to be disappointed when she can't stay on a restricted eating plan. By ditching popular diets and adopting an eating pattern that is sustainable, she can halt the weight gain and lower her blood pressure.

If your blood pressure is 140/90 millimeters of mercury (mm Hg) or higher (normal is 120/80 mm Hg), your doctor has probably diagnosed you with high blood pressure, although there is another classification, called prehypertension, when blood pressure is between normal and 139/89 mm Hg. High blood pressure, or hypertension, affects about 30% of Americans, and one in three adults has prehypertension. While most doctors prescribe a drug to treat high blood pressure and may advise cutting back on salt, sadly, many do not recommend an eating plan. The DASH diet has been shown to lower blood pressure by 8 to 14 points. For those with prehypertension, that means they might never develop high blood pressure. For those already diagnosed with hypertension, the DASH plan is the perfect eating style to keep your blood pressure from getting higher, and you may even be able to reduce the amount of medication you take.

The DASH plan is rich in fruits and vegetables, low-fat milk and dairy foods, whole grains, fish, poultry, beans, seeds, and nuts. It is lower in red meat, sweets, added sugars, and sodium. Researchers believe the key to lowering blood pressure is the combination of an eating pattern that is high in dietary fiber; rich in the minerals potassium, magnesium, and calcium; and lower in sodium. The DASH plan has two sodium levels: the traditional plan allows 2,300 milligrams (mg) of sodium per day and the lower-sodium version allows 1,500 mg. A typical US diet has about 3,400 mg of sodium. To give you a reference point, a teaspoon of salt has 2,300 mg of sodium.

The National Institutes of Health has developed free materials to help you follow the DASH plan. Sample meal plans at different calorie levels, recipes, and tracking forms are all available; see the Useful Resources section on page 68.

To get started on a DASH eating plan:

- Increase low-fat or fat-free dairy foods to three servings per day.
- Add a serving of vegetables to your lunch and dinner.
- Snack on fruit.
- Cut your meat portions to 6 ounces per day, about the size of two decks of cards.
- Eat a vegetarian meal once or twice a week.

Why It Might Work for You

Each year, the DASH plan is consistently ranked by *US News & World Report* as a "Best Diet" for healthy eating and for weight loss. This is the perfect plan for Caroline. She likes the structure of a meal plan, and with her recent diagnosis of high blood pressure, this plan can help her accomplish her twin goals of lowering blood pressure and losing weight. Here is a sample meal plan that Caroline can use to get started on the DASH plan:

Breakfast	Whole grain cereal, low-fat milk, strawberries, blueberries, coffee or tea
Snack	Nonfat-milk latte
Lunch	3 ounces of tuna on whole grain flatbread, dark leafy-green salad with olive oil and balsamic vinegar, fresh fruit salad, unsweetened ice tea with lemon
Snack	Apple, 1-ounce serving (about 23) of whole almonds, water
Dinner	Vegetarian meal of lentil and brown rice pilaf with pine nuts, grilled vegetables, mixed fruit salad, wine spritzer or sparkling water
Snack	Smoothie made with vanilla-flavored yogurt and frozen fruit

Flexitarian Eating Pattern

Georgia is a 64-year-old woman who is a regular at her 8 AM dance aerobics class. However, she feels like she is dragging halfway through the class. When asked about what she eats for breakfast, she says a cup of coffee. A self-described chronic dieter, Georgia eats a light lunch of green salad with fat-free dressing or a cup of fat-free, sugar-free yogurt. By the time dinner rolls around, she is starving, so she eats a big dinner with plenty of chicken or fish and green vegetables. She says she avoids red meat and starches, like potatoes or pasta, because she thinks carbs are fattening. Since she was so "good" all day at following her diet, she snacks in the evening and never misses dessert. Georgia has set up a vicious cycle of restricting food throughout the day and eating too much at night.

The name of this plan combines the words "flexible" and "vegetarian." You might think of it as vegetarian lite or vegetarian without the commitment to giving up meat, poultry, or seafood. It really is a plant-based diet. Dawn Jackson Blatner, a registered dietitian nutritionist who developed the plan, describes it this way:

> A Flexitarian diet is a vegetarian diet, but with flexibility. So because at its core it is plant-based eating, it naturally helps to decrease weight and the risk of chronic issues such as high blood pressure, high cholesterol, diabetes, and cancer. The flexibility of adding favorite animal-based foods occasionally, such as meat, poultry, and fish, increases the quality of life since it's easier to socialize, travel, and enjoy a wide variety of food.

This plan can help you move away from a meat-centered diet and explore other protein-rich options by discovering ways to enjoy a greater variety of whole grains and vegetables. The plan centers on fruits, vegetables, whole grains, herbs and spices (to flavor foods), and "new meats" (eg, protein-rich plant foods like tofu, beans, lentils, peas, nuts, seeds, and eggs). The basic plan calls for the following:

- 300-calorie breakfast
- 400-calorie lunch
- 500-calorie dinner
- Two 150-calorie snacks

The 1,500-calorie plan can be individualized for your activity level; most active adults will need more than 1,500 calories a day, but for those who are less active and want to lose weight, this is a good way to start. We like the idea of a flexitarian eating plan, but we also support vegetarian plans for those who choose to eliminate meat, poultry, or fish. Vegetarians tend to weigh about 15% less than meat-eaters, and even a flexitarian plan can result in lower body weight. Plant foods are nutrient rich yet filling, so a greater volume of food can be eaten without consuming excess calories.

Why It Might Work for You

We think this plan would work well for Georgia. It will give her the energy she needs and can help move her from her habit of eating the majority of her calories at night to spreading her calories throughout the day. This plan is also good for those who like to cook and experiment by seasoning foods with herbs and spices instead of just salt and pepper.

A flexitarian eating plan for Georgia might look like this:

Breakfast	One hard-boiled egg, steel-cut or old-fashioned rolled oatmeal with cinnamon and nutmeg, a tangerine, and coffee or tea
Lunch	Quinoa or other whole grain salad with mandarin orange slices, rice crackers, and water sweetened with fruit slices
Snack	Greek yogurt drizzled with honey and chopped walnuts
Dinner	Tofu noodle bowl with soba (buckwheat) noodles, bean sprouts, and carrots; vegetable egg roll; and sparkling, fruit-flavored water
Snack	Cottage cheese with diced pear and sunflower seeds and hot tea with lemon

Mediterranean-DASH Intervention for Neurodegenerative Delay (MIND)

Richard has read about the "miracle" of coconut oil on the internet. He says this superfood has powerful medicinal properties, and he also believes it can prevent Alzheimer's disease and is a potent anticancer agent. He has turned into the family chef and uses coconut oil in cooking, as a spread, and in smoothies. Richard is interested in eating well to support aging, and we applaud him for that. Unfortunately, coconut oil is not quite the miracle it is made out to be by its advocates. We think Richard should try another eating pattern to help preserve cognitive function.

A new dietary pattern to emerge in recent years is the MIND diet, which is based on research conducted at Rush University Medical Center in Chicago. Over 900 participants from retirement communities in the Chicago area were followed for 5 years; those who had the greatest adherence to the MIND diet suffered less cognitive decline. Because the MIND diet combines the best of the Mediterranean and DASH eating plans, researchers believe it can reduce cognitive decline and help to prevent Alzheimer's disease. There is strong evidence that certain dietary components have protective effects on the brain and cognition. The fats in fish (called omega-3 fats or fish oils), the B vitamins, vitamin E, and plant compounds called polyphenols can all affect brain function. Foods rich in these nutrients include seafood, green leafy vegetables, and berries. It is an exciting area of research, but the results should be considered preliminary, and there is no guarantee that following the MIND diet will prevent all cognitive decline or Alzheimer's disease. We include this plan because you will probably be hearing more about it as additional research results become available. MIND is an overall healthy eating plan that includes the foods we all should be eating—with an emphasis placed on brain-healthy foods—such as:

- Green leafy vegetables
- Nuts
- Berries
- Beans
- Whole grains
- Fish
- Poultry
- Olive oil
- Wine (but if you do not drink alcohol, you can still get the benefits from the other foods in the plan)

Why It Might Work for You

We like this plan, especially for Richard. He is interested in reducing his risk of Alzheimer's disease, yet he believes the hype around coconut oil. Despite the claims, there is no research to support using coconut oil to prevent Alzheimer's disease. While the evidence for the MIND diet's ability to prevent mental decline is promising, we look forward to seeing more results regarding this plan. Richard could use an oil change—from coconut to olive—for a proven health benefit. Following is what a typical meal plan would look like for Richard:

Breakfast	Bran cereal sprinkled with whole flax seeds and blueberries, with low-fat milk, coffee, or tea
Lunch	Wild rice salad with grilled salmon, wilted spinach with garlic and olive oil, and raspberry iced tea
Dinner	Large green leafy salad with sliced strawberries, avocado, sesame seeds, and strips of roasted chicken breast, dressed with an olive oil-based salad dressing; a whole wheat roll with olive oil; and water.
Snacks	Nuts and berries and iced green tea

Clarifying the Science on Macronutrients

The diet plans we recommend contain a healthy balance of the energy containing nutrients: carbs, proteins, and fats. Let's take a brief look at each macronutrient to clarify the science.

Carbohydrates

Carbs are the nutrient some people love to hate. How many times have you heard someone say, "I don't eat carbs"? What most people mean when they say that is that they don't eat starchy foods, such as bread or potatoes. We want you to rethink the role of carbs in your diet and recognize that carbs alone are not the fattening enemy. The key to a healthy relationship with carbs is choosing quality carbs and keeping portion size in check. Also, keep in mind that carbs are the best fuel for activity. Consider Georgia, whom we introduced earlier in this chapter. She didn't equate her inability to keep up in her exercise class to what she eats—or doesn't eat—in the morning. Georgia was simply running out of fuel. In the morning, after an overnight fast, the liver's storage of carbs (glycogen) can be nearly depleted. Breaking down liver glycogen in the early stages of exercise is a main source of fuel for working muscles, along with glycogen stored in muscle. So it is no wonder that Georgia is dragging during her aerobics class.

Different types of carbs are found in several food groups: grains (breads, cereals, rice, pasta), vegetables, fruit, and even some dairy foods. Carbs are generally classified as complex or simple, but even that classification is too simplistic. Complex carbs include both refined grains, such as white bread; whole grains, such as whole wheat bread; as well as the dietary fiber found in whole grains, vegetables, and fruit. Whole grains are the complex carbs we should eat more of. Sounds simple, right? But sometimes food labels make it tricky. For example, bread made from wheat flour isn't a whole grain food; the flour may come from a wheat grain, but when it's refined, its nutrient-rich bran and germ portions are removed. If you want a whole grain bread, choose one made with *whole* wheat flour or another whole grain; all three parts of a grain kernel, as shown in the image on the next page, must be used in a food for it to be considered whole grain.

Products labeled with terms like five grain, stone ground, or multigrain may contain whole grains, but they may not be 100% whole grain. Look for these words listed first in the ingredient list to ensure that you are getting whole grains:

- Whole wheat
- Barley
- Brown rice, wild rice, black rice, red rice
- Quinoa
- Bulgur
- Buckwheat
- Millet
- Whole sorghum
- Teff
- Triticale
- Whole oats

- Whole grain cornmeal
- Corn, including popcorn
- Whole wheat couscous
- Whole rye or rye berries

GRAIN ANATOMY

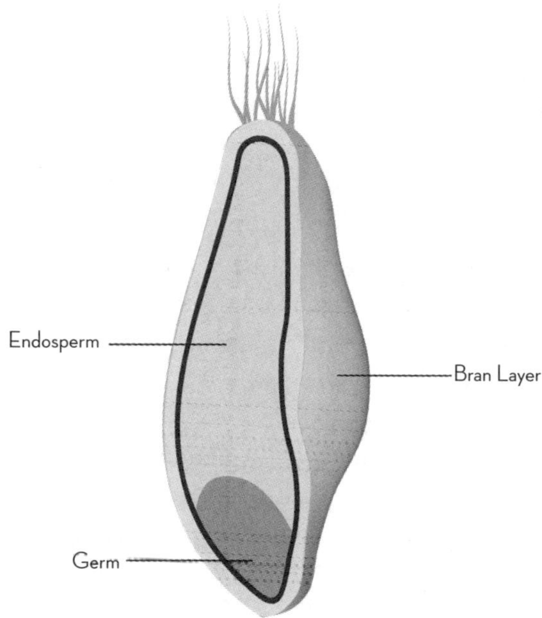

In addition to these whole grain ingredients, ancient grains are also making a comeback. Here are some less familiar whole grains that are worth trying.

- Amaranth
- Einkorn
- Whole farro
- Freekeh
- Kamut
- Spelt

Another reason to choose whole grains is for the dietary fiber. Fiber comes in two types. Most of us think of the insoluble type of fiber (the kind that can't dissolve in water) that our mothers referred to as "roughage." This type of fiber is mostly found in the bran portion of the grain kernel, and it is also in vegetables and in the skin of fruits. Insoluble fiber provides bulk in our stools and helps with regular bowel function. The other type of fiber is soluble fiber (that which dissolves in water to form a gel-like substance), which helps to slow digestion of foods and lower cholesterol and blood sugar. Most fruits and vegetables contain both insoluble and soluble types of fiber. Apples, for example, contain insoluble fiber in the skin and soluble fiber in the flesh of the fruit.

By now, you might be thinking, "But I love fragrant white jasmine or basmati rice with Asian food, but they aren't whole grains." You're right. They are not whole grains, but here is the good news: only half of grain intake needs to be from whole grains. Our advice is to eat mostly whole grains but enjoy other grains when a refined grain is preferred, like basmati rice with an Indian curry or long-grain white rice with red beans.

Vegetables are also rich in carbs, and for that reason, some veggies are maligned. Consider the poor potato. Potatoes are rich in many nutrients: B vitamins, vitamin C, potassium, and fiber. But potatoes often become less healthy when they're prepared or when they hang around with less-healthy company—think french fries, potato chips, and gobs of butter or sour cream on a loaded baked potato. Enjoy potatoes in their natural form: baked potatoes served easy on the toppings and with the skin intact or mashed potatoes or potato salad with the skin still on for a "dirty" variety of a favorite potato dish to make it more nutrient rich.

Simple sugars, another type of carb, are found in various foods, including sugar-sweetened beverages, most desserts, cookies, candies, pastries, fruit, and milk products. We should all be trying to eat less *added* sugar, but this doesn't include the naturally occurring sugar found in fruits and dairy products. The natural sugar in fruit comes with water, vitamins, minerals, and fiber, so don't fret over the sugar content in fruit. The same is true with dairy; it naturally contains the sugar lactose, which may not taste sweet but is considered a simple sugar. Proposed changes to food labels include listing added sugars, but, for now, naturally occurring and added sugars are lumped together. With the current nutrition label, for example, it is hard to determine how much of your yogurt contains natural sugar from the milk versus added sugars from fruit or sweetened flavoring. The label examples shown below illustrate the US Food and Drug Administration's proposed label changes to highlight sources of sugars.

We see a disturbing trend of positioning some sugars as healthier than others. This includes cane sugar, honey, brown sugar, agave, coconut sugar, and raw sugar (note that sugar sold as "raw" is just slightly less processed than table sugar; it isn't really raw in the strict sense of the word). Except for the sugars in fruit and dairy, sugar is

CURRENT NUTRITION FACTS LABEL (LEFT) AND PROPOSED NEW LABEL SHOWING ADDED SUGARS (RIGHT)

Nutrition Facts

Serving Size 2/3 cup (55g)
Servings Per Container About 8

Amount Per Serving	
Calories 230	Calories from Fat 72
	% Daily Value*
Total Fat 8g	**12** %
Saturated Fat 1g	**5**%
Trans Fat 0g	
Cholesterol 0mg	**0**%
Sodium 160mg	**7**%
Total Carbohydrate 37g	**12** %
Dietary Fiber 4g	**16** %
Sugars 12g	
Protein 3g	
Vitamin A	10%
Vitamin C	8%
Calcium	20%
Iron	45%

* Percent Daily Values are based on a 2,000 calorie diet. Your daily value may be higher or lower depending on your calorie needs.

	Calories:	2,000	2,500
Total Fat	Less than	65g	80g
Sat Fat	Less than	20g	25g
Cholesterol	Less than	300mg	300mg
Sodium	Less than	2,400mg	2,400mg
Total Carbohydrate		300g	375g
Dietary Fiber		25g	30g

Nutrition Facts

8 servings per container
Serving size 2/3 cup (55g)

Amount per serving	
Calories	**230**
	% Daily Value*
Total Fat 8g	**10%**
Saturated Fat 1g	**5%**
Trans Fat 0g	
Cholesterol 0mg	**0%**
Sodium 160mg	**7%**
Total Carbohydrate 37g	**13%**
Dietary Fiber 4g	**14%**
Total Sugars 12g	
Includes 10g Added Sugars	**20%**
Protein 3g	
Vitamin D 2mcg	10%
Calcium 260mg	20%
Iron 8mg	45%
Potassium 235mg	6%

* The % Daily Value (DV) tells you how much a nutrient in a serving of food contributes to a daily diet. 2,000 calories a day is used for general nutrition advice.

Reprinted from the US Food and Drug Administration.

sugar. Many sugars have a health halo because they sound more natural or might contain a trace of nutrients, but don't be fooled. Your body cannot distinguish between the different types of sugars. Try to eat less of all added sugars, especially from sugar-sweetened beverages because these calories can add up very quickly. Examples of some of the sugars you might find on a food ingredient label are listed to the right.

Examples of Sugars Found in Ingredient Lists

Sucrose (table sugar)
Glucose (also called dextrose)
Fructose (also called levulose)
Maltose
Brown sugar
Molasses
Honey
Beet sugar
Confectioner's or powdered sugar
Raw sugar
Turbinado sugar
Agave nectar
Maple syrup
Cane sugar
Sugar-cane syrup
High-fructose corn syrup

Why We Need Carbohydrates

Carbs are the body's preferred fuel for muscles and the brain. Carbs are carried in the blood as glucose and stored in the muscles and liver as glycogen. Both are readily available to use when needed. However, during periods of inactivity, it is easy to overconsume carbs, and excess carbs are then stored as body fat. Getting enough carbs is important, because without carbs, the body breaks down protein. If there is no spare protein because it is all being used for fuel, there is no protein left to be used to build or maintain muscle or to perform the other critical functions of protein.

Protein

If carbs are the nutrient some people love to hate, then protein is the nutrient they love to love. Proteins are made up of small units called amino acids. Twenty amino acids are needed in the diets of healthy adults, and nine of those amino acids are essential, meaning the body can't make them—so it's essential to get them from the foods we eat. In terms of their protein quality, foods are frequently classified as "complete" (meaning they contain all nine of the essential amino acids in the amounts needed to support health) or "incomplete," meaning the food does not contain all nine essential amino acids. Below is a list of food sources of complete and incomplete proteins.

Complete Proteins	Incomplete proteins
Meat (beef, pork, lamb)	Nuts and seeds
Poultry (chicken, turkey, duck)	Grains
Fish and seafood	Vegetables
Eggs	Pulses (beans and peas)
Dairy (milk, cheese, yogurt)	
Soy foods	
Quinoa	

A food that supplies incomplete protein doesn't make it a poor choice; it just means it doesn't contain all of the essential amino acids. When you eat a variety of foods with incomplete proteins throughout the day, what one food lacks in essential amino acids, another may provide. Take rice and beans, for example. This tasty dish found around the globe in many varieties illustrates the value of consuming foods containing complementary proteins: the amino acids in short supply in rice are complemented by the amino acids in beans, making it a good protein-rich dish. Whether they're consumed at the same time, as is the case with rice and beans, or at different meals during the day, their proteins complement each other and are considered complete.

Most protein-rich foods contain more than just protein. In fact, many of our favorite protein-containing foods can also provide a hefty dose of fat. For example, a 3-ounce cheeseburger made with ground beef labeled as 70% lean and a slice of American cheese has 28 grams of protein but also 22 grams of fat, which can be about one-third of your daily fat allowance, depending on your calorie needs. That is why we encourage meat eaters to consume only lean meat.

The amount of protein needed every day may not be as much as you might think. The Recommended Dietary Allowance (RDA) is 0.8 grams of protein per kilogram of body weight or 0.4 grams of protein per pound of body weight. As we age, however, consuming more protein is beneficial to maintain and build muscle mass (see Chapter 6 for more about getting enough protein). Consider these food choices for a vegetarian: 2 scrambled eggs, whole wheat toast with peanut butter, a handful of almonds, lentil soup, a tofu noodle bowl, an apple, and rice crackers. At first glance you might think only the eggs, nuts, and tofu provide protein, but when you add it all up, this vegetarian's intake contains about 72 grams of protein, a sufficient amount for a person who needs about 1,600 to 1,800 calories per day.

The other aspect of protein nutrition that is emerging as a top concern is distributing protein throughout the day. Most of us backload our protein: we eat a lot of protein at dinner and smaller amounts at breakfast and lunch. We discuss protein in more detail and will show you how to evenly distribute protein across your meals in Chapter 6.

Why We Need Protein

First, let's clear up some possible confusion. Most people understand that protein is a nutrient we need every day, and most people can identify foods that provide protein. The confusing part for some people is that when protein-rich foods are consumed, our bodies break down the protein from our food into individual amino acids. Our cells then reassemble those amino acids into the tens of thousands of different proteins needed for the body to function. For example, protein is a component of or plays a role in the following:

- growth of muscles, bones, skin, hair, nails, and connective tissue (like ligaments and tendons);
- prodution of enzymes that make all chemical reactions in the body happen;
- production of hormones that regulate everything from glucose entry into cells (insulin) to stimulating appetite (ghrelin);
- transportation of compounds like oxygen and iron through the blood;
- well-being of immune system components;
- regulation of acid-base and fluid balance; and
- supply of last-ditch energy source.

Note that we referred to protein as a "last-ditch energy source" because, under normal conditions, carbs and fat do a great job of providing us with energy. But when carbs or fat are in short supply, protein can also be broken down to provide energy. It is better to let protein do its important jobs, however, and leave energy production to the carbs and fats.

Fat

Fat is the most energy (calorie) dense of all the nutrients; it has more than twice as many calories as carbs or protein. But before you decide to cut calories by cutting out fat, think again. There are different kinds of fat. Some are healthier than others. And no one can deny the special sensory qualities of fat, which make some foods taste so good. The creamy taste of ice cream just isn't the same when the fat is removed, and the smell of bacon sizzling in a frying pan tempts most everyone.

A great deal of controversy surrounds dietary fats and blood fats (lipids). One day the news is reporting that fat is bad, and the next you hear that butter or bacon are health foods. Remember what we said in the beginning of this chapter: science evolves. The complex relationship of dietary fats and the subsequent risk of heart disease is still being untangled, but we know a few things for certain:

- All fats have the same number of calories, but some fats are better for you than others.
- Simply classifying fats as "bad" or "good" doesn't tell the whole story. Within the bad fat group, some of the fats are neither good nor bad when it comes to health risk. And when we classify a fat as good, that doesn't mean it is the only fat you should eat or that you can eat as much of it as you want.
- Heart disease is still the leading cause of death for men and women in the United States, and looking at ways to reduce your risk will always involve diet—and watching fat intake.

Fats can be classified in many ways, but for our purposes, we will group fats by their health-related properties. Examples of foods that supply the different types of fats are included in the box on page 57.

- Plant sources of fat are generally considered healthy because they tend to have favorable effects on blood lipids. Oils extracted from olives, sunflowers, soybeans, rapeseed (canola oil), corn, flax seeds, safflowers, walnuts, and peanuts all supply healthier fats, including monounsaturated and polyunsaturated fats. They all have different taste profiles, and some are better for different cooking applications than others, but they are all healthy oils. The exceptions to the rule are tropical oils (palm, palm kernel, and coconut), which are less healthy than the other plant oils because they can increase our blood cholesterol levels and contribute to inflammation.
- Whole foods that are high in total fat but contain healthy fats include avocados, peanuts, tree nuts (such as almonds, pistachios, walnuts, pecans, brazil nuts, hazelnuts, and pine nuts), and seeds (such as flax, sunflower, and pumpkin). Fatty fish also contain healthy fats, such as omega-3 fats, which is the reason for the recommendation to consume a few meals with fish each week. Not every fish contains healthy fats, but cold-water fish, such as salmon (farmed or wild), Albacore tuna, herring, mackerel, and (while not a fish) scallops, are good choices. Fish like tilapia, cod, or grouper are great sources of protein but don't contain much of the healthy fats.
- Fats that are less healthy, called saturated fats, are found in tropical oils, lard, butter, stick margarine, and shortening. Saturated fats are usually solid at room temperature, and although most have a negative effect on blood cholesterol levels and increase the risk of heart disease, some saturated fats do not. An example is chocolate; the fat in chocolate is a type of saturated fat that is considered neutral, which means it doesn't raise or lower blood cholesterol levels. Enjoy chocolate in moderation, keeping in mind that it is not a health food and is still high in sugar and calories. Another emerging area of research concerns the fat in milk and cheese. It may be that dairy fat, when consumed in the matrix of milk or cheese, doesn't have a negative effect on blood lipids and health.

- *Trans* fat is a type of fat that has been significantly reduced in today's foods, and with good reason; it has been shown to be a major player in heart disease risk. *Trans* fats are fats that are changed in food processing (called hydrogenation), where the molecule is flipped, like those Transformers your kids used to play with, making the fat less healthy than other fats. If you see the words "partially hydrogenated" in the ingredient list on a food label, this means that the food contains some *trans* fats.

Type of Fat	Examples of Food Sources
Saturated fats	Shortening, some stick margarine, butter, full-fat dairy foods, beef and ground beef, sausage, bacon, some bakery items (like cookies, pastries, croissants), hydrogenated fats, coconut and palm oils
Monounsaturated fats (also called omega-9 fats)	Olives, olive oil, avocados, nuts, canola oil
Polyunsaturated fats (also called omega-6 fats)	Oils or soft-tub margarines or salad dressings made with corn, soybean, safflower, sunflower, and canola oil
Polyunsaturated fats (also known as omega-3 fats) Omega-3 fats include: • alpha-linolenic acid (ALA) • eicosapentaenoic acid (EPA) • docosahexaenoic acid (DHA)	Flax seeds and oil, walnuts, and fatty fish, like salmon and tuna
***Trans* fats**	Some bakery foods contain *trans* fats, but most have been removed
Cholesterol	Only found in animal-based foods: meat, fish, eggs, dairy fats

Why We Need Fat

Fat is an essential nutrient, just like protein and carbs. Fat also plays an important role in our bodies, even though most of us would like to do with a little less of it. We need fat for:

- Cell membranes, which use it to help keep some substances out and let others in, sort of like a cell gate keeper
- Brain function (more than 50% of our brain is fat)
- Transporting vitamins A, D, E, and K, which are classified as fat-soluble nutrients
- Its role as a component of the systems that control blood thickness and blood pressure
- Protecting our delicate internal organs with a layer of padding

Certain fats, like certain amino acids, cannot be produced by our bodies and must be obtained from what we eat. Fat in our diet provides two of these essential fatty acids: alpha linolenic acid (an omega-3 fatty acid found in flax seeds and some vegetable oils, like canola oil) and linoleic acid (an omega-6 fatty acid found in vegetable oils). Most fat-containing foods contain a mixture of saturated and unsaturated fats; very few are 100% of one type of fat, as illustrated in the comparison of dietary fats show below.

Comparison of Dietary Fats

Dietary Fat

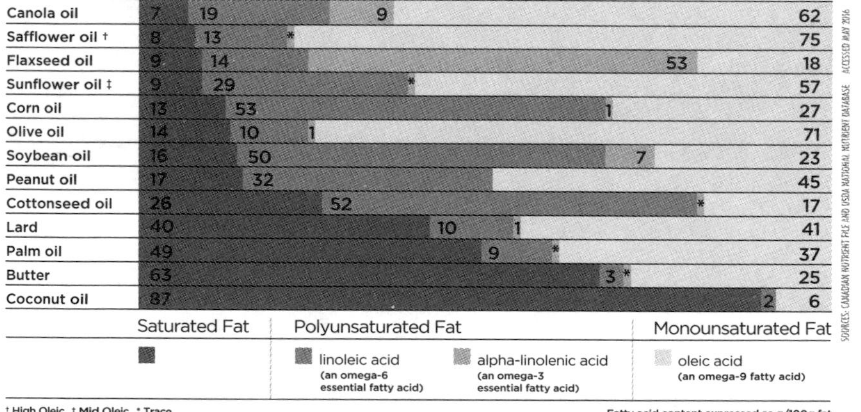

Reprinted with permission from the Canola Council of Canada

Confronting Myths About Healthy Eating

MYTH: Never eat white foods.

REALITY: There's no need to exclude white foods. Cauliflower, onions, garlic, potatoes, mushrooms, and white fish are all healthy white foods. The logic behind this sentiment usually refers to avoiding white flour and white sugar, both of which are refined products. Eat more whole grains and less sugar, but don't judge a food by its color. Remember, the key words are "eat less," not "never eat." We wouldn't want you to miss out on enjoying a piece of your grandchild's birthday cake!

MYTH: Sugar is toxic and addictive.

REALITY: Chronic high sugar intake is linked to many chronic diseases, including obesity and cardiovascular disease, but sugar isn't toxic according to the definition of the word: something that is poisonous or deadly. Nor is it addictive, like a drug. When people say they are "chocoholics," they don't have a physical addiction—maybe they have a strong psychological pull to the food, but not an addiction. Sugar-rich foods stimulate pleasure, but that doesn't equate to toxicity or addiction.

MYTH: Sugar substitutes are poisons that trick your brain into eating more, thereby causing obesity.

REALITY: Sugar substitutes (also called artificial sweeteners, nonnutritive sweeteners, or low-calorie sweeteners) are far better studied than dietary supplements. The Academy of Nutrition and Dietetics position paper on sweeteners says, "All [nonnutritive sweeteners] approved for use in the United States are determined to be safe." A recent systematic review of both animal and human studies concluded that sugar substitutes do not increase calorie intake or body weight. The balance of evidence indicates that using low-calorie sweeteners in place of sugar can lead to lower calorie intake and body weight. Note the emphasis of "in place of"—drinking a diet soda with a rich chocolate dessert is not going to help with weight loss or controlling blood sugar.

MYTH: Bread is fattening.

REALITY: Any food can be fattening if you eat too much of it, as it can bump up your daily calorie intake to a level that's beyond than your daily needs. Bread is one of the foods that many people restrict because it is easy to overeat. When you are in a restaurant, do you always dive into the bread basket and ask for refills? If so, bread may indeed be fattening. But there is no reason to eliminate bread from a healthy eating plan when you keep your portions in check. And whole grain breads supply important nutrients, like fiber, B vitamins, and minerals.

MYTH: No one should eat red meat.

REALITY: While many of the eating plans we recommend suggest eating less red meat, you can enjoy a steak or burger on any of the plans. The key to choosing red meat is moderate portions (3 or 4 ounces) and lean cuts (cuts with "loin" or "round" in the name). Red meat is nutrient rich: it contains quality protein, B vitamins (niacin, B-6, and B-12), selenium, zinc, and iron. Vitamin B-12 is needed in greater amounts as you age, and it is only found in animal foods.

MYTH: A high-protein diet causes kidney disease.

REALITY: A higher protein intake causes the kidneys to work slightly harder to filter urea, the waste product produced from protein. But it is the kidneys' job to filter waste, a job that healthy kidneys do quite well; high-protein diets do not overly stress the kidneys or cause kidney disease. A person diagnosed with kidney disease might be told to follow a lower protein diet, but protein did not cause the disease.

MYTH: Soy foods should not be eaten by those who have had breast cancer.

REALITY: Fear of eating soy for breast cancer patients was driven by the presence of isoflavones (also called phytoestrogens), which are found in soy foods. Isoflavones are similar in structure to a form of estrogen, but isoflavones are not estrogen. Research shows that the ways isoflavones affect the body are distinct from the effects of estrogen. Small differences in structure can greatly affect the activity of a compound in the body. The American Cancer Society and the American Institute for Cancer Research reviewed the existing research on the soy–cancer connection and concluded that breast cancer patients can safely consume up to three servings of soy foods a day. Eating soy foods is not associated with increased cancer risk for those with breast cancer or those who have had breast cancer. Overall, consumption of soy foods does not prove dangerous for breast cancer patients; they can experience and utilize the benefits of soy as part of a healthy, active lifestyle.

Commonly Asked Questions About Eating for Optimal Aging

Is the Paleo diet a healthy eating plan?

The Paleolithic (Paleo), or caveman, diet is based on the idea that early men and women ate wild game, wild plants, roots, and berries and that those foods are therefore best for the body. Even though the life expectancy of early humans was not very long compared with modern folks, Paleo diets are popular with many fitness enthusiasts and are sometimes advocated for weight loss. The Paleo diet includes lower-fat animal proteins like bison, grass-fed organic beef, lamb, and pork. It also encourages consumption of lean chicken, turkey, and wild-caught fish. Roots, wild greens, and nonstarchy vegetables, as well as some nuts, seeds, and berries that were foraged by early humans, are also allowed on the diet. The foods not included are grains, potatoes, pulses, peanuts and peanut butter, dairy foods, and processed meats like luncheon meats, bacon, hot dogs, and fast-food burgers. The plan includes some healthy foods, but it is also restrictive and might be difficult to follow in the long term. It also may be lacking in essential nutrients typically supplied by these eliminated foods.

Can a vegetarian diet be healthy for older adults?

A vegetarian diet can be healthy at any age. We did not include this as one of our recommended plans because it might be too restrictive for some, and only about 2% of adults over the age of 65 practice vegetarianism. There are many types of vegetarians—from strict vegans who eat no animal products to lacto-ovo-vegetarians who eat dairy foods ("lacto") and eggs ("ovo"). Or you may simply choose to be a part-time vegetarian, or flexitarian, and enjoy meatless meals regularly. Vegetarians who eat a variety of vegetables, grains, fruits, nuts, seeds, and legumes have nutritionally adequate diets. The Academy of Nutrition and Dietetics recognizes that vegetarians tend to be at lower risk for many chronic diseases, including heart disease, high blood pressure, type 2 diabetes, obesity, and some types of cancer. The key to reaping the benefits of vegetarianism is to include the healthy foods mentioned here; simply eliminating meat won't make you a healthy vegetarian.

Should older adults avoid processed foods?

The term "processed food" has become synonymous with "unhealthy." However, think about this: canned black beans, yogurt, peanuts, and baby carrots are all processed in some way, so these foods would fall in the category of processed foods. Yet we think you would agree that they are all healthy foods. To make it even more confusing, there is no clear-cut definition for processed food. Instead of generalizing that all processed food is bad, base your choices on the food's ingredients and nutrients. Eat less of foods that contain added sugars, refined grains, sodium, and saturated fats, but don't think that you must mill your own flour or bake your own bread to eat healthy.

What does eating chocolate in moderation really mean? Is dark chocolate healthier than milk chocolate?

While there is no official definition of moderation when it comes to eating chocolate, about an ounce or two of chocolate a couple of times a week seems moderate. When cocoa (also called cacao) beans are processed to make chocolate, the level of healthy compounds, called flavonols, decreases. Dark chocolate is more likely to contain the healthy flavonols than milk chocolate, but don't overlook other foods, such as cherries, apples, and black and green tea to get flavonols. Chapter 4 provides more information on plant compounds with healthy properties.

Should older adults be eating probiotic foods for gut health?

One of the hottest topics in health and wellness is the gut microbiome. The human gastrointestinal tract, which plays host to one of the most complex ecosystems on earth, contains more than 100 trillion microorganisms. Probiotic means "for life." While there are many claims regarding the benefits of probiotic foods and beverages, the two benefits supported by the strongest science are their roles in a healthy digestive tract and a healthy immune system. Some foods, beverages, and dietary supplements contain bacteria that promote a healthy gut microbiome, such as *Bifidobacterium* and *Lactobacillus*. The foods with the highest amounts of live active cultures of these good bacteria are those that are naturally fermented, like yogurt. The International Scientific Association for Probiotics and Prebiotics recommends daily intake of 10^9 colony-forming units (a way to count the bacteria content) of probiotics, which can be achieved through consuming approximately 1 cup of yogurt. To get a variety of probiotics, choose yogurts and other products containing added (or fortified with) probiotics, such as kefir. Look for the "Live & Active Cultures" seal on products to determine whether they contain probiotics.

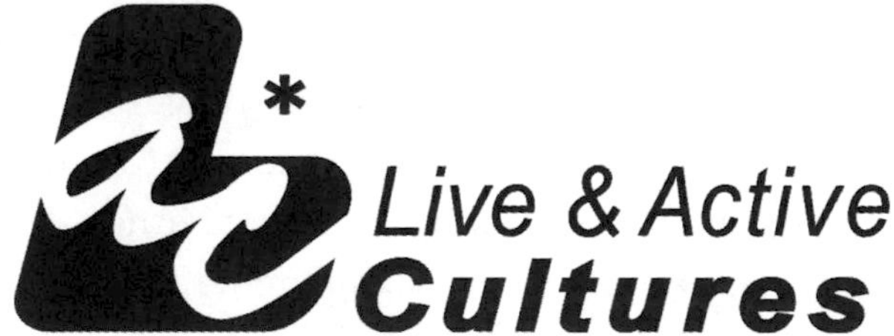

Reprinted with permission from the National Yogurt Association (NYA)

While many people are aware of probiotics, prebiotics get less attention but are equally important. Prebiotics selectively stimulate growth of good bacteria. Probiotics help to establish the gut microbiome, and prebiotics feed it. Prebiotic sources include carbohydrate-rich foods that contain compounds that cannot be digested because we lack the enzymes to do so. The gut microbiome ferments carbs into energy and other nutrients. Prebiotic foods include artichokes, asparagus, banana, chickpeas (garbanzo beans), garlic, honey, leeks, oats, and onions. Prebiotics are also added to foods as functional ingredients, and one of the foods that has been most closely studied to determine its prebiotic effect is chicory root fiber, which is also called inulin.

Having the Confidence to Make Eating Patterns Work for You

As we age, we may think that what we eat doesn't much matter anymore and that the damage is done. But just as with exercise, healthy eating can begin at any age. Eating healthy has many benefits, regardless of your age, including gaining more energy to get you through the day; reducing your risk of developing the most common chronic diseases of aging; controlling your weight; supporting the demands of exercise; and providing your body with the needed nutrients to repair and renew skin, muscle, bone, and every body system. As we have presented, there are multiple eating patterns that promote optimal aging. After reviewing the plans, one might be seem more appealing than another, but you might also decide to adopt certain features of more than one plan and create your own, and that is fine too. We found that the experts we talked to in our Conversation with an Expert sections don't advocate rigid adherence to a specific plan but rather try to make healthy choices about what to eat, when to eat, and how to eat to support your health goals and fitness routines. We suggest that you take a look at your usual intake and then tweak it to make improvements. An example of making small changes to a daily menu to offer health benefits is shown on the next page.

Meal	Current Food Choices	New Food Choices	Benefits
Breakfast	Bagel, cream cheese, and coffee	Mini whole wheat bagel with peanut butter, banana, and coffee	Increased fiber and protein and an additional serving of fruit
Lunch	Fast-food cheeseburger meal with french fries and a soft drink	Fast-food salad with grilled chicken and water with sliced lemon	Increased fiber; leaner protein source; and decreased calories, fat, and sugar
Dinner	Beef and bean burrito with nachos and cheese sauce and a large margarita	Handful of tortilla chips with salsa and guacamole, a bean burrito with a side of rice and beans, a small margarita, and water	Increased healthy fat and decreased saturated fat and meat by substituting plant-based protein; fewer calories from alcohol
Dessert	Ice cream with chocolate cookies	100-calorie ice cream novelty	Decreased calories and sugar
Snacks	Potato chips Pretzels	8 ounces of yogurt with a serving of nuts	Increased healthy fats and fiber, improved satiety, and the addition of a probiotic food

Conversation with an Expert

> The diversity of our gut microbiome changes as we age, and the deviations are not going in a healthy direction. The number of beneficial bacteria decrease dramatically, and the number of pathogenic bacteria increase. These changes coincide with parallel changes in immune function and greater susceptibility to disease as we age.

So says Jo Ann Tatum Hattner, MPH, RD, a registered dietitian nutritionist with a master's degree in public health. She is the coauthor (with Susan Anderes) of *Gut Insight: Probiotics and Prebiotics for Digestive Health and Well-Being*. As she approaches 75, Jo Ann has a targeted strategy to keep her gut healthy: "In my refrigerator, you will always find yogurt, kefir, and fermented foods for populating the gut with healthy microbes and vegetables and fruits with prebiotic fibers," she says. (A comprehensive list of prebiotic food sources can be found on her website gutinsight.com under [also listed in the Useful Resources on page 68]). Jo Ann includes gut-healthy foods in all her meals and describes her typical diet as follows:

> In the morning, I eat oatmeal with raisins (prebiotic fiber sources). For lunch, my gut-health foods include fresh or frozen fruits and vegetables, as well as fresh greens or celery, which I have in a salad with added protein. Or I might use the fruits and vegetables to make a smoothie with kefir or a probiotic supplement. I often cook dinner by first sautéing garlic, shallots, or onions (prebiotic fiber sources) in olive oil and then adding fish, chicken, or lean meat. I serve them accompanied by grains and fresh vegetables with prebiotic fibers like asparagus or artichokes.

She also advocates fermented foods, like sauerkraut, as side dishes for their gut-healthy bacteria. In addition to developing and maintaining a healthy gut microbiome, she stays physically active by walking, swimming, riding a stationary bike, practicing yoga, and weight training. She says she is motivated to exercise "because both physical health and brain health can be enhanced by physical activity. Getting my heart rate up promotes optimal blood flow to the brain. And I know that as we age, we lose muscle mass, so activities that build muscle are mandatory." Jo Ann recommends that we all develop a target food list that contains gut-healthy foods; shop for fresh foods, especially produce; cook; and enjoy a meal with friends or family. "I expect researchers will find that by keeping our gut microbe population healthy with foods containing natural live cultures and by feeding these beneficial microbes with prebiotic fibers, our microbes will help protect us against many of the chronic diseases that are more prevalent as we age," Jo Ann adds.

How the Authors Eat for Optimal Aging

We enjoy eating and try to eat a varied diet without depriving ourselves of any particular food.

Chris: I make sure to eat a protein and whole grain-rich breakfast five or six mornings every week. That means eating a custom mix of whole grain cereal with additional high-fiber cereal topped with protein-enriched milk and some berries. One or two days a week, I enjoy a veggie-laden omelet with a toasted English muffin or bagel. Breakfast helps get me through morning exercise classes and keeps me feeling full until lunchtime. While not everyone agrees that breakfast is the most important meal of the day, it is for me because it includes important nutrients, like protein, calcium, vitamins D and B-12, and dietary fiber, all of which are needed in greater amounts as we age. I include two servings of dairy foods every day, usually yogurt for probiotics and one additional calcium-rich food, like a serving of almonds. I don't follow any particular meal plan, but a combination of all of the meal plans presented in this chapter works best for me and my husband. I enjoy cooking, trying new recipes, and finding ways to lighten up a recipe. I get together with several friends for a bimonthly supper club to try new recipes and enjoy meals together. And even though I live in the South, I rarely eat fried foods and never drink sweet tea, but that is more personal preference than for health reasons.

Bob: I don't follow a specific diet plan, but I try to eat a varied diet of healthy foods and beverages on most days so that I don't need to worry about occasionally consuming foods and beverages that some might consider less than healthy. I know that the contents of the cupboards and refrigerator at home play a major role in what I grab to eat as a quick meal or snack, so I'm very happy that my wife makes plenty of healthy choices available for me.

Useful Resources

Academy of Nutrition and Dietetics (www.eatright.org)

▻ *Tips, articles, and advice on many topics related to healthy eating for all ages*

Flexitarian Diet (https://dawnjacksonblatner.com/books/the-flexitarian-diet)

▻ *Information on following this eating plan found in the book,* The Flexitarian Diet: The Mostly Vegetarian Way to Lose Weight, Be Healthier, Prevent Disease, and Add Years to Your Life. *New York, New York: McGraw-Hill; 2009.*

Global Organization for EPA and DHA Omega-3s (http://goedomega3.com/consumers)

▻ *Information on the health benefits of omega-3 fats*

Grain Foods Foundation (http://grainfoodsfoundation.org)

▻ *Health information, including videos, on including grains in your diet*

Gut Insight (http://gutinsight.com)

▻ *Information on prebiotics and probiotics*

National Heart, Lung, and Blood Institute (www.nhlbi.nih.gov/health/health-topics/topics/dash/ and www.nhlbi.nih.gov/health/resources/heart/hbp-dash-week-dash-html)

▻ *Description of the DASH eating plan and a sample weekly eating plan*

National Yogurt Association (http://aboutyogurt.com)

▻ *Tips to help identify healthy strains of bacteria in yogurt*

Oldways (https://oldwayspt.org/traditional-diets/mediterranean-diet)

▻ *Tips and sample foods and menus for following a Mediterranean diet*

US News & World Report (http://health.usnews.com/best-diet)

▻ *Evaluations of the "best" diets based on different conditions and goals*

CHAPTER

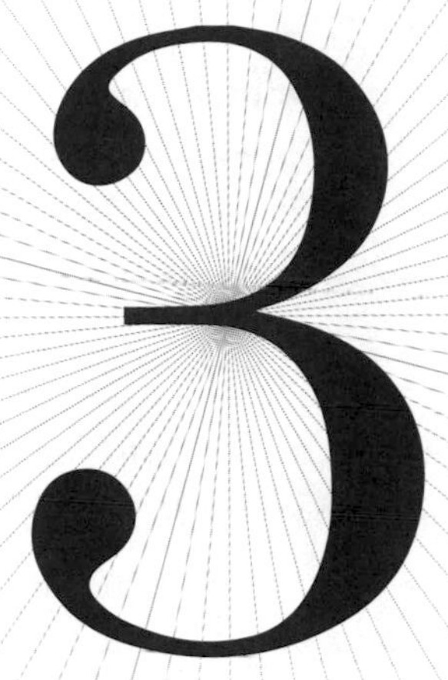

STAYING WELL HYDRATED

The Bottom Line

There's no doubt that it can be easy to forget about drinking enough during the day, and if you're one of those people, we think you'll be pleasantly surprised by how much better you'll feel once you begin to meet your daily fluid needs. Fortunately, staying well hydrated is fairly easy to accomplish; doing so simply requires being aware of how much fluid you need on a daily basis and then changing your hydration habits accordingly. This chapter will help you assess and address your daily fluid needs. Here are some key points to keep in mind about hydration:

- Mild dehydration can be common as we age, and this strains the body's ability to function normally.
- During typical everyday activities, mild dehydration is easily tolerated, but when coupled with physical activity or warm weather, dehydration limits your ability to function optimally.

- **With illness or hospitalization, dehydration can complicate treatment, prolong recovery, and even increase the risk of death.**
- **Daily fluid needs depend on our body size, physical activity level, and environment.**
- **As a general guideline, women should consume about 8 cups of water and other beverages each day, and men about 12 cups. Remember that food also contributes to your fluid intake.**

Rick is a 59-year-old, healthy, active, and hard-working man. He likes to keep constantly busy until he runs out of energy at the end of each day and falls asleep on his couch watching television. As the owner of a small manufacturing company, Rick's hectic workdays include extended periods of time when he is sitting at his desk or in meetings, along with frequent short walks into his manufacturing shop to talk to employees and troubleshoot projects. Rick likes to exercise early in the morning and sometimes again after work. He's devoted to his fitness routine and attacks each workout with the same enthusiasm and dedication he expects of himself during each workday. Rick rarely takes a day off from his super-sweaty workouts and feels guilty when he does. He prides himself on his competitive nature and his ability to keep up with or surpass the physical capabilities of much younger men. Yet more often than he'd like during workouts, and even during some workdays, Rick runs out of steam, both physically and mentally. The occasional headaches, lightheadedness, and muscle fatigue he experiences are, in his opinion, nuisances that are all part of a hard-charging lifestyle. Rick doesn't realize that his body needs periodic rest days to fully recover from and adapt to his exercise routine. In addition, his sweaty workouts combined with hectic workdays make it tough for him to stay well hydrated. The combination of dehydration and insufficient recovery saps his physical and mental energy.

Introduction

The human body is basically a leaky bag of water with legs. We're leaky because we are constantly losing water and electrolytes (also called minerals or ions). Unless we're sweating, we're usually not aware that we're losing water. Even so, we are constantly losing fluid. For example, our kidneys are continually producing urine that slowly accumulates in our bladders, water molecules steadily seep through our skin (a process different from sweating), our bowel movements contain water, and additional water is lost in the humidified air of each and every exhalation. Those sources of water loss typically amount to anywhere between 70 to 110 ounces (the equivalent of 9 to 14 cups, or 2 or 3 liters) each day, depending upon our body size, activity level, and the temperature and humidity of the environment.

We lose fluid constantly but only consume fluid periodically, hence the challenge of staying well hydrated. And when we are completely hydrated, that condition lasts only a short time. Our hydration status naturally rises and falls throughout each day as we lose and replace fluids. Rick often sweats every day of the week during his workouts and on the job, so his daily fluid needs may be in excess of 150 ounces (the equivalent of 19 cups or 4.5 liters.) If that sounds like a lot of fluid, that's because it is. Let's assume that Rick has to drink 80% of that volume, with the remaining 20% coming from the food he eats: 80% of 150 ounces is 120 ounces (15 cups). If Rick is awake 16 hours during the day, he would have to drink about 1 cup of liquid every waking hour to replace the fluid lost from his body. On days when he sweats more, he'll have to drink more to keep up; on days he sweats less, his fluid intake can fall accordingly.

Keep reading to learn more about why hydration is so important and how to calculate your own daily fluid needs.

ASSESS YOURSELF: IN REVIEW

Stop and take the Assess Yourself quiz on the next page before continuing on.

After reviewing your responses, you may already recognize a few changes you'd like to make in your daily drinking habits. For exam-

Assess Yourself: Hydration

What is usually the first thing you drink in the morning? And what is usually the last thing you drink at night?

- ☐ Water
- ☐ Coffee
- ☐ Soft drink
- ☐ Tea
- ☐ Juice
- ☐ Milk
- ☐ Other

After getting out of bed in the morning, how much time elapses before you have something to drink?

- ☐ Less than 30 minutes
- ☐ 30 minutes to 1 hour
- ☐ Greater than 1 hour

What volume of fluid (ounces) do you consume at that first drinking occasion (1 cup = 8 fluid ounces)?

- ☐ A sip (a few ounces)
- ☐ Less than 1 cup (up to 8 ounces)
- ☐ More than 1 cup (more than 8 ounces)

How much additional fluid do you consume in the morning before lunch? Include coffee, tea, soft drinks, fruit juice, milk (including on your cereal), water (bottled and tap), etc.

- ☐ Less than 2 cups (16 ounces)
- ☐ 2 to 4 cups (16–32 ounces)
- ☐ More than 4 cups (32 ounces)

How much fluid do you typically consume at lunch?

- ☐ None
- ☐ 1 cup
- ☐ More than 1 cup

How much fluid do you consume between lunch and dinner?

- ☐ Less than 2 cups (16 ounces)
- ☐ 2 to 4 cups (16–32 ounces)
- ☐ More than 4 cups (32 ounces)

How much fluid do you consume after dinner and before bedtime?

- ☐ Less than 2 cups (16 ounces)
- ☐ 2 to 4 cups (16–32 ounces)
- ☐ More than 4 cups (32 ounces)

What is the total volume of the preceding values (in cups or ounces)?

____

How many times during a typical day do you urinate?

- ☐ One or two
- ☐ Three or four
- ☐ More than four

How many times do you wake to urinate during the night?

- ☐ None
- ☐ Once
- ☐ Twice or more

Do you often wake up thirsty?

- ☐ Yes
- ☐ No

ple, if you drink one or more cups of coffee to start each day and don't eat much until later in the morning, you are prolonging the time that you are at least mildly dehydrated and shortening the number of hours during the day that you have to catch up. The same is true if you simply don't have much to drink at breakfast. Do you take advantage of all the possible drinking occasions throughout each day, or do you find yourself getting so busy that you often forget to drink something between breakfast and lunch or between lunch and dinner? Are your trips to the bathroom infrequent, and is your urine a strong yellow color and of small volume? Producing about 3 ounces of urine (a volume of less than ½ cup) each hour is normal, so when you do go to the bathroom, you should have a general sense of how much urine you are losing. Do you wake up once each night to urinate? Doing so is definitely a nuisance, but it's also a sign that you are adequately hydrated. Do you frequently wake up thirsty? If so, that's a sign of dehydration and should be a reminder to start drinking.

Clarifying the Science on Hydration

Why Is Hydration So Important?

Water is the most biologically important molecule in the body because water molecules are involved in virtually every function of the body, from individual cells and organs to every system in the body. The importance of water to our health should be obvious from the simple fact that the majority of our body weight is comprised of water. For the first 6 months of our lives, we are 75% water, a value that gradually decreases and hovers around 60% for most of our lives. As we age and lose muscle mass, that value can fall further—to around 50%. Keep in mind that muscle and many other tissues are roughly 75% water, a value that doesn't change much as we age. Not surprisingly, fat is only 10% to 40% water, so the more fat we store, the lower our total body water level is.

Water plays some obvious roles in our bodies, such as being the primary constituent of most cells and blood; in short, all of the countless molecules in our bodies are dissolved in water. But the importance of water goes far beyond this. Among its many roles in the body, water is a lubricant that enables all movements, a shock absorber that cushions our every step, and a coolant that keeps us from overheating, making water central to life in about every way imaginable. No other nutrient is needed in as a large a quantity or as often as we need to consume water. Our physical, mental, and emotional well-being all depend on staying well hydrated.

The US Institute of Medicine offers guidelines for daily water as part of the Dietary Reference Intakes (DRIs). These intake guidelines for vitamins, minerals, and water are determined by a group of experts who study the scientific literature and make recommendations supported by research studies. In the chapter on water, the experts recommend a daily water intake for adults of 2.7 liters (the equivalent of 11 cups or 91 ounces) per day for women and 3.7 liters (the equivalent of 15.5 cups or 125 ounces) for men. Keep in mind that these recommended amounts include the fluids you consume from water, other beverages, and from foods, and they represent daily intakes that sit right at the median for the thousands of people in the database used by the experts. In other words, half the people in the database need less fluid each day and half need more. This means that you may need more or less than 2.7 or 3.7 liters (11 to 15.5 cups) each day. In reality, our fluid needs vary from day to day, depending on our activity level and environment. Common sense and science both dictate that we should drink more on days when we sweat and a little less on days when we don't.

How the Body Controls Hydration

Because we are constantly losing water (the many routes to water loss listed in the box on the opposite page show how it can be difficult to stay hydrated), it makes intuitive sense that our bodies are equipped with ways to make sure we replace what we've lost. Thirst is one way to ensure that we recognize and act on the need to replace lost water. The other way the body controls hydration is by varying urine production. When the body senses that it has too much water on board, the kidneys increase urine production; when we're dehydrated, our kidneys reduce urine production. Special sensors throughout our bodies constantly monitor the consistency and volume of blood, altering thirst and urine production accordingly.

In simple terms, dehydration reduces the volume of our blood and increases its saltiness. Small changes in those two measures quickly invoke a wide array of responses that spark thirst and reduce urine production. For that reason, whenever your urine is of small volume, is dark yellow, and smells distinctively like urine, there is a very good chance that you're dehydrated. Under normal conditions, a urine volume of about 3 ounces (100 milliliters) per hour is healthy. Of course, that value will be less in smaller people and more in larger people. Urine production declines when we sleep, so that total urine output over 24 hours is typically about 50 to 85 ounces (1.5 to 2.5 liters). For those who sweat often and therefore need to consume more fluid during the day, urine production ramps up accordingly. In fact, in some laborers, soldiers, and athletes, daily urine production can be in excess of 300 ounces (2.5 gallons; 10 liters).

Water Loss
Urine
Feces
Insensible loss through skin
Breathing (exhaling)
Sweating (exercise, fever)
Metabolism
Saliva
Vomiting
Diarrhea
Lactation
Menstruation

Water Gain
Beverages
Foods
Metabolism

Factors that Influence Hydration

The good news is that, compared with our younger selves, our older selves usually do a good enough job eating and drinking throughout the day to maintain proper hydration, thus minimizing the health risks associated with dehydration (summarized in the next section). But if we're not careful, dehydration can quickly become a problem. For example, simply contracting a common cold or flu is enough to reduce thirst and appetite for days, making temporary dehydration a likely outcome that makes us feel worse and recover more slowly. Any circumstance that increases fluid loss challenges our hydration status. Living in a warm climate and physical activity of any sort that works up a sweat are obvious ways we lose more water.

Brian couldn't wait to move to Florida after he retired from his job as an insurance agent in Michigan's Upper Peninsula. He and his family vacationed regularly in Florida and grew particularly fond of the state's southwest coast, with its beaches and lush vegetation. A vacation week or two each year fueled Brian's desire to make that area home after their retirement. And that's exactly what they did, settling into a retirement community between Fort Myers and Naples. Brian recalled a few occasions during vacations when he, his wife Lois, and their two kids struggled with the heat and humidity, but it was a small price to pay for time away from the constant chill of a Michigan winter. When Brian and Lois began living full time in Florida, however, the periodic stretches of high heat and humidity drove them into their air-conditioned home for days on end. At times, the sweltering heat was almost too much to bear; it seemed too hot for even short walks in the neighborhood, let alone for a round of golf. They hadn't moved to Florida to stay indoors, but being outside on hot days was uncomfortable and exhausting. Unfortunately, staying inside makes it more difficult to cope with the heat because the body does not have a chance to adapt—or acclimate—to the hot weather. If Brian spent time outside each day, working up at least a little sweat, he'd soon be better able to cope with the heat.

As older people gravitate to warmer climates, getting accustomed to the heat and humidity is important for their day-to-day comfort and their new lifestyle, health, and even longevity. In Brian's case, neither he nor his wife had become acclimated to their new environment, preferring instead the comfort of air conditioning. When we're not acclimated to the heat, even short journeys outside can feel overwhelming. In addition, for anyone with heart problems or other serious illnesses, exposure to the heat is a major stress that can sometimes be too much for a weakened heart.

We're all aware that heat waves are associated with an increase in deaths, particularly among out-of-shape and frail, elderly individuals. The vast majority of those deaths, however, aren't from heat stroke but from heart failure. Whenever we're exposed to the heat, our bodies are programmed to increase the volume of blood that circulates in the skin to aid in heat loss. For anyone with compromised heart function and perhaps reduced blood volume from dehydration, heat stress can overwhelm the heart's ability to pump blood, possibly resulting in heart attack and death. To acclimate to the heat we must spend time outdoors, gradually building our tolerance over a 10- to 14-day period. Specifically, that means spending at least 90 minutes each day in the heat, doing our normal physical activities. Yes, we'll be uncomfortable for the first few days, but as our bodies adjust, we'll become more and more comfortable. Scientists refer to this as improved thermal comfort, and it's one of many adjustments our bodies make as we become heat acclimated. Other benefits include an enhanced capacity for physical activity and reduced overall strain on our bodies. The combination of heat exposure and physical activity promotes the full benefits of acclimation.

The rate at which people acclimate to the heat varies widely. Some acclimate within a couple of weeks, while others are resistant to acclimation and require more time. As we acclimate to the heat, our sweating begins sooner and ramps up faster. We stay cooler as a result, but we lose even more water as sweat. Fortunately, one of the benefits of heat acclimation is that we become better drinkers, drinking more often and in greater volume. An added benefit of heat acclimation is that cellular changes occur to protect us against stressors associated with cardiovascular disease and other maladies. This added protection, called cross-adaptation, is one of the reasons why regular physical activity helps reduce the risk of so many health problems.

Other factors that can influence our hydration status are exposure to altitude, consumption of alcohol, and prescription medications. Whenever we go to altitudes above 5,000 feet, urine production increases and appetite is diminished, setting the stage for dehydration, headaches, and fatigue. After a few days, those symptoms subside, but it's always a good idea to pay extra attention to hydration whenever we travel to high-altitude destinations. As most of us know from experience, alcohol consumption also increases urine production, making it more difficult—but definitely not impossible—to stay well hydrated. In fact, beverages of all sorts contribute to hydration. While shots of hard liquor are an exception to that rule, beer, wine, and mixed drinks all contain enough water to contribute to hydration. The medications we take can also affect our hydration status—and vice versa. Diuretics that stimulate urine loss and laxatives that promote bowel movements result in increased fluid loss. Dehydration is also associated with taking antihistamines, blood pressure medications, and chemotherapy. In addition, dehydration increases the potency of medications—an important reason to make sure we consume adequate fluid throughout each day.

Hydration, Health, and Disease

Stella is an 82-year-old grandmother of eight who lives alone and busies herself with household chores, periodic visits with friends, church activities, and occasional meals and social events with nearby family. Though she was an avid gardener in her younger years, Stella's arthritis and gradual loss of muscle mass have reduced her physical activity to little more than what's required for daily living. She tries to avoid getting up during the night to urinate and has found that if she doesn't drink anything after 7 PM, she can usually sleep through the night uninterrupted. Stella would like to have the energy to accomplish more during the day but has concluded that slowing down is just what happens to everyone as they age. In Stella's case, not drinking anything after 7 PM increases the chance that she'll become dehydrated, a condition that can contribute to her feelings of low energy. Her decision to stop drinking early in the evening extends the hours in which her body dehydrates, making it more difficult for her to make up the difference during the day.

As we age—and especially when we have to deal with periodic illnesses, broken bones, and disease—staying well hydrated helps us feel better, both physically and mentally. Dehydration is linked with an increased risk of falling, confusion, kidney stones, urinary tract infections, and constipation, along with an increased risk for bladder and colon cancer. Research also shows that being dehydrated even increases the frequency of driving errors. We all dehydrate as we sleep because our kidneys are constantly producing urine and because we lose water with each exhalation. In other words, we all wake up weighing a little less than when we went to sleep because of that water loss.

Staying well hydrated is clearly good for our health. Perhaps just as important as its roles in reducing the risk of diseases and disorders, being well hydrated gives us more energy to enjoy life. Sometimes being down in the dumps, feeling irritable, and having low energy can all be caused by dehydration. Simply drinking more and restoring body fluids might be all it takes to snap out of those doldrums.

It's also important to keep in mind that many adults are dehydrated on admission to the hospital, complicating treatment and increasing morbidity (sickness) and mortality (death). Aside from not drinking enough during the day, many older adults take diuretics and laxatives, which increases water loss and makes maintaining normal hydration more challenging. As mentioned before, dehydration quickly increases the strain on our cardiovascular system, stressing the heart's capacity to pump blood. It's no wonder that we don't feel good when we're dehydrated.

But how do we know when we or a loved one is actually dehydrated? Each and every day, we dehydrate and rehydrate on an ongoing basis. That's normal. But prolonged dehydration is not. Unfortunately, there's no simple way of determining if someone is truly dehydrated, aside from a hospital blood test. However, there are a few signs to look for:

- dizziness, especially upon standing
- unusual weakness or fatigue
- apathy
- irritability
- dry armpits
- sunken eyes
- dark yellow or brownish urine of smaller volume than normal
- dry mouth
- greater thirst than usual (or sometimes absence of thirst)
- rapid weight loss from one day to the next

If many of these signs are present, there's a good chance dehydration is the cause. Of course, if weakness and dizziness persist even after consuming more fluids, it's a good idea to consult your doctor.

A side benefit of increasing daily water intake is that even small increases in water consumption are associated with reductions in calorie intake. In other words, having an extra glass of water—especially before a meal—can help fill you up and support weight loss efforts. The next time you think you are hungry or thirsty for a soft drink or alcoholic beverage, try drinking water first. Often that's enough to temporarily satisfy hunger or thirst and reduce subsequent calorie intake.

Confronting Myths about Hydration

MYTH: Dehydration is always bad.

REALITY: All of us tolerate low levels of dehydration periodically each day, so in that regard, dehydration isn't a noticeable issue. Problems arise when dehydration becomes more pronounced and prolonged, and when we are physically active, exposed to hot weather, or ill. All things considered, it's always better to be well hydrated than to be dehydrated.

MYTH: Water is the best hydrator.

REALITY: Water is definitely a good hydrating beverage, especially when it's consumed along with foods. The sodium and other minerals (ions, electrolytes) we ingest when we eat food help keep water in our bodies. However, consuming plain water without food quickly turns off our thirst mechanism and turns on urine production, so we actually drink less and lose more liquid. One reason why sports drinks contain electrolytes is to help maintain the desire to drink and reduce urine production during exercise. Other beverages, such as flavored waters, juices, milk, tea, coffee, and soft drinks, all count toward your daily fluid intake. The key is choosing beverages that you like to drink but also being mindful of the calories that often come with drinks.

MYTH: Caffeinated drinks dehydrate.

REALITY: Caffeine is a very mild diuretic, so mild that over the course of a day it has little impact on our overall hydration. That's particularly true for those who are regular coffee, tea, and cola drinkers and have become accustomed to daily doses of caffeine. For those who don't consume much caffeine, urine production will increase modestly, but subsequent fluid intake will be more than enough to offset those small urine losses.

MYTH: You can't have too much water.

REALITY: Actually we can, and the results can be deadly. This cautionary tale is an example of how too much of a good thing can be a very bad thing. Consuming far too much water in a short period of time causes the sodium level in our blood to plummet. When that happens, water from the blood passes into the brain, causing the brain to swell, sometimes so severely that seizures, coma, or death may result. That condition is known as *hyponatremia*—abnormally low blood sodium concentration. It is a fairly rare occurrence but one that has claimed the lives of athletes and others who have ingested very large volumes of water over a few hours. We all periodically consume too much fluid, and when that happens, our kidneys excrete the excess as urine. As long as our kidneys are healthy, we can handle this excess fluid. There's no need to worry about hyponatremia unless unusually large volumes are being ingested. For example, gulping down a couple quarts of fluid in an hour or over-drinking for many days can cause blood sodium levels to fall to dangerous levels. In other words, it's aberrant drinking behavior that can be dangerous.

MYTH: Water comes only from beverages.

REALITY: In the United States, we typically consume about 20% of our daily water intake in the foods we eat. For example, bananas are roughly 75% water by weight, a hot dog is 50%, and even a chicken breast is 65% water, unless it's cooked to a crisp.

MYTH: I need to drink 8 cups of water each day.

REALITY: This errant advice was initially intended to be a simple way for people to identify the minimum volume of fluid to consume each day. Eight cups of water amounts to 64 ounces or 2 quarts, roughly the minimum volume of water required for a sedentary person each day. Unfortunately, some people misunderstood that advice and thought they had to drink 8 cups of water each day, on top of all their other fluid intake from beverages and foods, when the reality is that daily fluid can come from a combination of water, other beverages, and foods.

MYTH: If I'm not thirsty, I'm not dehydrated.

REALITY: That sounds logical, because we know thirst is the body's way to prevent problematic dehydration. However, dehydration itself is what causes us to become thirsty in the first place. In other words, by the time we're thirsty, we're already slightly dehydrated. That's usually not much of a problem, except for when lots of sweat is being lost during exercise. Dehydration impairs exercise performance and increases the risk of heat illness, so sweaty athletes are advised to drink regularly and to start drinking before they become thirsty, with the goal of minimizing weight loss (that is, minimizing dehydration).

MYTH: Clear urine is a sign of good hydration.

REALITY: Clear urine is not normal. Your urine color should be more like lemonade than like apple juice, but crystal-clear urine is one sign that we may be drinking too much. Urine is colored because of its primary contents, which include urea; a variety of minerals; and creatinine, a by-product of energy metabolism. Certain foods and medications can change urine color (red beets can give urine a reddish hue, B vitamins can give urine a vibrant yellow color, asparagus may cause a greenish color, and certain antibiotics can result in orange-colored urine). Urine color is a general indicator of hydration status, but dilution with toilet water sometimes makes it difficult to determine its actual color. Keep in mind that if your urine appears to be dark yellow and is of smaller volume than usual, you may be dehydrated. Simply drink a glass of water or another beverage to help get you back on track.

MYTH: Beer dehydrates.

REALITY: An old saying goes that beer doesn't stay in us long enough to change color, and it's true that all drinks containing alcohol increase urine production. In more scientific lingo, we'd say that ethanol (the alcohol part of alcoholic beverages) is a moderately potent diuretic. But beer is mostly water, and if we consume beer with salty foods, such as chips and pizza, its diuretic effect is lessened. In fact, most alcoholic beverages can contribute to our daily hydration needs, provided we don't overdo it. The exception is that shots of any hard liquor are far more dehydrating because they deliver very little water and a lot of alcohol. Also true is that some hangover effects are due to dehydration, making it all the more important to avoid drinking too much alcohol in the first place.

MYTH: Special detox waters aid in removing toxic elements from the body.

REALITY: The notion that we can drink special beverages that detoxify the body is understandably very appealing. After all, who wants a toxic body? The truth of the matter is that our intestines, liver, and kidneys are well equipped for the job of detoxifying the bloodstream. Special drinks can't help. Urine and feces remove unwanted, unneeded, and dangerous compounds and elements from the body. Staying well hydrated certainly helps all of those functions, but detox waters don't provide any additional benefits.

MYTH: Alkaline water prevents the body from becoming too acidic.

REALITY: Claims for alkaline waters include an ability to boost metabolism, improve nutrient absorption, and slow the aging process, all supposedly because alkaline waters neutralize acids in the bloodstream. There's no doubt at all that the body has to maintain a fairly tight balance between acidity and alkalinity (referred to as pH). Fortunately, our bodies have a number of different ways to accomplish this balance, which rely on our blood, lungs, and kidneys. Unless we are gravely ill, consuming alkaline water, or even infusing it directly into the bloodstream, has no effect or benefit beyond just staying well hydrated. Most commercial alkaline waters have a pH (a measure of acidity and alkalinity) that is close to 7.0, the value associated with neutral pH. The body is well equipped to maintain the pH of its various fluid compartments so that they don't become too acidic or too alkaline; as a result, drinking alkaline water is unlikely to make much impact. In fact, stomach fluid (gastric juice) is naturally very acidic to aid in digestion, while the fluid contents of the small intestine are closer to neutral pH, as is blood. It would take an enormous volume of alkaline water to change the pH of any of those spaces.

Commonly Asked Questions About Hydration

Should older adults drink sports drinks?

Conventional sports drinks can be a great way to stay well hydrated during any physical activity that causes sweating. Sports drinks contain carbohydrates (sugars) and electrolytes (minerals) that stimulate rapid fluid absorption and sustain hydration. Older adults who really push themselves during workouts or competitions can benefit from sports drinks for hydration, as they supply energy to exercising muscles. Don't confuse sports drinks with energy drinks; the latter are not formulated for exercise and often contain high levels of carbohydrates, caffeine, and other ingredients.

Is drinking plain water good for weight loss?

Yes, having a glass of water before meals can reduce the number of calories you consume and, in that way, aid weight loss. And, of course, drinking water instead of any beverage that contains calories can help satisfy thirst and avoid unneeded calorie intake.

Are there any advantages to filtered water, spring water, mineral water, or other special waters?

Not surprisingly, water is water, regardless of its source. What differs from one water to another are the substances—solutes—dissolved in the water. It's obviously wise to avoid consuming water that is contaminated with potentially harmful chemicals, but the small amount of minerals contained in clean tap, bottled, and mineral waters do not constitute a health risk or benefit. The best approach is to consume whatever water tastes best to you.

Having the Confidence to Make a Hydration Plan Work for You

The National Institutes of Health recommends that older adults consume a full cup of water whenever they take medicine; consume fluid before exercise or going outside on a hot day; and take sips of water, juice, or milk between bites of food at meals. That's all good advice for people at any age, but it tells us nothing about the volume of fluid each of us should consume.

As mentioned earlier in the chapter, the US Institute of Medicine suggests that adult women drink 2.7 liters (note that a liter equals 1.06 quarts, so the numbers are about the same if you prefer to think in quarts) each day and that adult men should strive for 3.7 liters. Those suggestions are helpful in that they give us a ballpark idea of how much fluid we may need, but all of us are different in that regard. A small, sedentary, 85-year-old woman who spends her days in an air-conditioned home may need only 2 quarts of fluid each day to maintain her hydration, while a larger man of the same age, living in a warm climate and spending hours each day outside, may need twice that volume or more to stay hydrated. To muddy the waters even further, his hydration needs won't be 4 quarts every day but will vary, depending in large part on how much he sweats.

To give you an idea of how daily fluid needs can be met with water and other beverages—and the inherent challenge in doing so—the table on the next page illustrates how often and how much fluid has to be consumed to meet fluid intakes of 2, 3, and 4 quarts per day.

In short, there is no tried-and-true way to determine how much fluid we need. But there are ways to estimate our needs, establish what seems like a reasonable minimal volume to ingest each day, and follow that recommendation to see how we feel. A variety of smart

FLUID INTAKE

	2 quarts/day*	3 quarts/day*	4 quarts/day*
Breakfast	12 ounces	20 ounces	24 ounces
During the morning	10 ounces	12 ounces	20 ounces
Lunch	12 ounces	20 ounces	24 ounces
During the afternoon	10 ounces	12 ounces	20 ounces
Dinner	12 ounces	20 ounces	24 ounces
During the evening	8 ounces	12 ounces	16 ounces

*Assuming that an additional 20% of daily fluid intake is provided by water in foods

phone apps can help make those determinations easy. Take a look at the box below for some examples of hydration apps, or search the App Store (iPhone iOS operating system) or the Google Play Store (Android operating system) for other options. Some of the apps include established behavioral-change techniques to help us create new and sustainable drinking behaviors.

EXAMPLES OF HYDRATION APPS THAT TRACK DAILY DRINKING BEHAVIOR

iPhone

Drink Water Reminder
iDrated
Splashy Water Tracker
Watango
Water Alert
Water Log
Waterlogged
Water Tracker Daily

Android

AddWater Pro
Aqualert Water Reminder
Gulp
My Water Balance
Water Alert Pro
Water Balance Hydration Tracker
Water Minder
Water Tracker

Conversation with an Expert

Larry Kenney, PhD, is a long time professor and researcher at Penn State University. More specifically, Larry is the Marie Underhill Noll Chair in Human Performance and a professor of physiology and kinesiology. One of Larry's areas of scientific expertise is hydration in older adults, a topic that is becoming increasingly personal as Larry recently turned 60. Larry's in-depth understanding of the challenges that people—especially active people—face in staying well hydrated throughout the day gives him insights most people don't have about the benefits of staying hydrated. Not one to follow a rigid diet or obsess over what he eats and drinks, Larry makes sure he ups his fluid intake on days when he sweats. He says:

> As I've become older, I am more conscious of wanting to stay physically active well into my 90s! Because of several knee surgeries, I focus my aerobic exercise on walking. To maintain strength and flexibility, I do weight training (low resistance, multiple reps) three times each week. Both of those activities help with my passion—playing competitive golf.

While most older adults don't lose large volumes of sweat on a regular basis, changes that occur as we age can make staying well hydrated even more of a challenge. Larry explains:

> As we age, our ability to match our thirst to our fluid needs diminishes, and our kidneys' ability to conserve fluid may likewise decrease. So it's a good idea to simply think about "drinking ahead of thirst" on those days when you know you'll be active and sweating. Being out all day in the heat, whether you're hiking, gardening, golfing, or hanging out at the beach, can lead to dehydration if you don't consider your fluid needs.

How the Authors Stay Hydrated

Chris: In a typical day, I drink filtered water because my house is supplied with well water, so filtering it makes it taste better. Black coffee is my go-to morning beverage. I also drink calcium-fortified orange juice or cranberry juice with breakfast. In the summer, I like lime-flavored sparkling water and unsweetened black, green, or ginger iced tea. I carry a 16-ounce water bottle to exercise classes to stay hydrated when working out. In general, I steer clear of sugar-sweetened beverages because I don't want the liquid calories.

Bob: I've never liked the smell or taste of coffee, so orange or tart cherry juice is my go-to morning beverage, along with milk or hot chocolate. I try to drink a mix of beverages throughout the day to make sure I keep up with my hydration needs, especially on days when I exercise. And, of course, it's tough to turn down a beer when it's offered, but only if I can have pizza or chips along with it to supply the sodium needed to minimize the diuretic effect! And about once each month, I rely on a hydration app on my phone to chart my daily fluid intake. Doing so always reminds me that I need to drink more often, especially on busy days.

Useful Resources

Academy of Nutrition and Dietetics (www.eatright.org)

▷ *Tips, articles, and advice on many topics related to hydration as it relates to healthy eating for all ages*

American College of Sports Medicine (www.acsm.org/docs/brochures/selecting-and-effectively-using-hydration-for-fitness.pdf)

▷ *Information on selecting and effectively getting enough hydration for physical activity*

Centers for Disease Control and Prevention (www.cdc.gov/healthywater/drinking/nutrition/index.html)

▷ *Basic information on the importance of meeting daily fluid needs, along with links to other resources related to fitness and nutrition*

Cleveland Clinic (http://my.clevelandclinic.org/health/diseases_conditions/hic_avoiding_dehydration)

▷ *Helpful, practical information about how to avoid dehydration*

National Institute on Aging (www.nia.nih.gov/health/publication/whats-your-plate/water)

▷ *Advice on hydration, including a video on getting enough to drink*

Tufts University: MyPlate for Older Adults (http://hnrca.tufts.edu/myplate/myplate-for-older-adults/fluids)

▷ *Tips on staying well hydrated, along with a list of high-water-content fruits and vegetables that can help with daily hydration (and good nutrition)*

CHAPTER

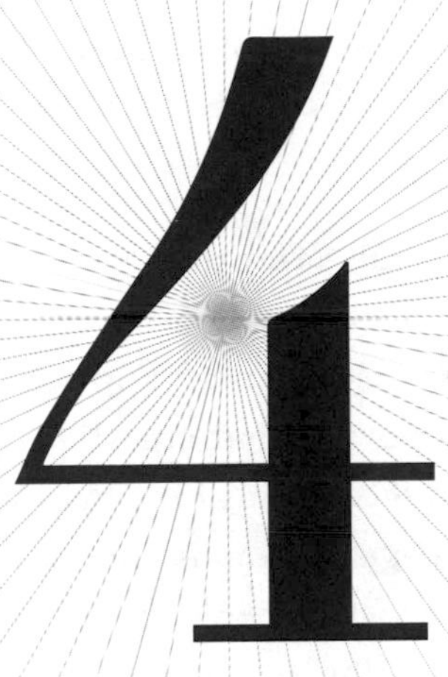

VITAMINS, MINERALS, PHYTONUTRIENTS AND SUPPLEMENTS

The Bottom Line

Vitamins, minerals, and plant compounds called phytonutrients (plant nutrients) play a role in hundreds of processes that prevent disease and promote good health. Vitamins were originally identified in foods as the substances that cured deficiency diseases. Vitamin C, for example, is chemically known as ascorbic acid, named for its scorbutic role—that is, its role in curing and preventing a deficiency disease called scurvy. The word vitamin comes from the words vital amine, chosen because scientists first thought these compounds were amino acids, the building blocks of proteins. We've come to realize that they are their own special class of nutrients. It has also become clear that there's more to vitamins than preventing deficiency diseases and that, in fact, vitamins play many roles in maintaining optimal health.

Minerals also have many functions in the body and are essential to maintain bone health, blood pressure, and blood sugar, along with many bodily processes. Phytonutrients are the compounds found in plants that protect the plant from diseases. They are being studied for a host of healthy properties. Here are some key points to keep in mind:

- Vitamins and minerals are called micronutrients because they are needed in small amounts.
- Phytonutrients are found in a variety of plant foods and have many healthy properties that are still being discovered. There are no recommended intakes for phytonutrients at this time.
- The best ways to get vitamins, minerals, and phytonutrients are by using spices when cooking and eating a varied diet that includes plenty of colorful fruits, vegetables, beans, nuts, seeds, and whole grains, as well as low-fat or fat-free dairy foods and lean meats, poultry, and fish.
- Eating foods that contain vitamins, minerals, and phytonutrients provides a health synergy that you don't get from taking dietary supplements alone.
- Nutrients that may fall short in the diets of those over the age of 50 include vitamins A, C, D, and E and the minerals calcium and magnesium.
- Dietary supplements can help you get nutrients that are in short supply in your diet; evaluate your usual dietary intake and use supplements to fill any gaps.
- More isn't better when it comes to vitamins and minerals; most have a level designated as the Tolerable Upper Limit (or UL) that indicates how much is too much when taking dietary supplements

---

This chapter will introduce some terms that might be new to you; definitions for these terms can be found on the next page.

Term	Definition
Antioxidant	A substance that inhibits or stops oxidation; dietary antioxidants include vitamins C and E, as well as the mineral selenium
Carotenoid	A pigment in plants that give, them color; carotenoids are a type of phytonutrient found in carrots, pumpkin, squash, and many other deeply colored fruits and vegetables
Free radical	In chemistry, an unpaired electron that results from oxidation; if left unchecked, it can lead to cell damage
Heme iron	The form of iron found in animal foods; better absorbed than iron from plant food sources
Micronutrient	A nutrient, such as a vitamin or mineral, that is needed in small amounts
Nonheme iron	The form of iron found in plant foods; not as well absorbed as the iron from animal-based food sources
Oxidation	A chemical reaction that occurs when something is exposed to oxygen; it can occur quickly or over time. A sliced banana turning brown when exposed to the air is an example of a quick reaction, whereas metal rusting is a result of long exposure to oxygen in the air
Phytonutrient	A nutrient that has disease-preventive and disease-fighting properties; also known as plant chemical or plant compound ("phyto" means plant)
Prooxidant	A substance that promotes oxidation; iron is a nutrient that acts as a prooxidant
Recommended Dietary Allowance	The amount of daily intake of a nutrient recommended to avoid a dietary deficiency of the nutrient
Senescence	The aging process; the opposite of adolescence
Shortfall nutrient	A nutrient that a specific age group is not consuming enough of, as determined by national food intake surveys
Synergy	Two or more things working together to produce a combined effect that is greater than separately
Tolerable Upper Limit	Abbreviated UL, highest level of intake of a nutrient possible that has no adverse risk to health

Candice freely admits that she doesn't like vegetables or most dairy foods. When she was young, her mother served canned asparagus, canned green beans, and canned carrots, and Candice found their texture and taste unappealing. She jokes that most of her foods come from the "beige" food group: bagels, bread, rice, chicken breast, potatoes, and bananas. At a recent physical, her doctor inquired about her calcium and vitamin D intakes and suggested a bone density test. Candice has always maintained a healthy weight and is approaching her 60th birthday. She wonders if her limited food choices negatively affect her health and wants to know if it is too late to change her eating habits. Candice isn't unusual in that she is stuck in a food rut, always eating the same few foods without exploring new foods or cuisines. A lifetime of low-nutrient food choices can have a negative effect on many body systems as the years add up.

Introduction

Although they're needed in very small amounts, micronutrients have a big impact on health. Vitamins and minerals are essential to almost every function in the body; some have structural functions (such as building and maintaining bone, teeth, and muscle) and some have regulatory functions (assisting in all chemical reactions in the body, maintaining water balance, and protecting cells from wear and tear, to name but a few). Phytonutrients are neither vitamins nor minerals, but they play important roles in health maintenance and disease prevention.

The need for vitamins and minerals is based on age and gender, and for most nutrients, there are guidelines to help us determine how much is needed. Earlier in the book we talked about the Recommended Dietary Allowance (RDA) for vitamins and minerals. In addition, most vitamins and minerals have a UL. These values, which are set by a group of experts, provide guidance on how much of a nutrient is needed to prevent deficiency. Note that the RDA is the *recommended* dietary allowance; not a required daily amount. The goal is to include foods that provide the needed nutrients close to the RDA over the span of a few days; there is no need to hit the target 100% every day to be healthy. The UL value is another important piece of information that suggests how much is too much, especially for those who use dietary supplements. It is difficult to reach the UL with foods, but it can be easy to exceed it with supplements.

No RDAs or ULs have been set for phytonutrients, and researchers are still learning about the more than 20,000 compounds in plants and how they may afford protection from disease. Much of the research revolves around cancer prevention and how phytonutrients may alter or halt changes in cells that lead to cancer. The American Institute for Cancer Research advocates for a diet that is two-thirds plant based (fruits, vegetables, whole grains, pulses, nuts, and seeds) for cancer prevention. A combination of foods that contain vitamins, minerals, fiber, and phytonutrients may offer a nutritional synergy that a single food or supplement can't provide.

As we age, our need for vitamins and minerals changes; for some nutrients, more is needed, and for others, less. More isn't always better for vitamins and minerals, in part because they work together for good health. Overloading one nutrient can cause a decrease in another, so it is a balancing act to get enough, but not too much, of all the nutrients we need.

Vitamins, minerals, and phytonutrients go by many names, and the terminology can be overwhelming. Instead of presenting a detailed list of each nutrient, we are taking a functional approach by grouping nutrients to help you understand why they are needed, along with naming good food sources for each. We know you don't go to the store with beta carotene, ascorbic acid, or folate on your shopping list, so we will translate the nutrients into food choices to help you become more aware of what foods are rich in vitamins, minerals, and phytonutrients. Don't fear ingredients that are hard to pronounce. Food is actually made up of many chemical-sounding substances. For example, you might be concerned about eating a food with ferrous sulfate, but that is just the chemical name for iron that may be added to a food. How about thiamine mononitrate? This is a form of vitamin B-1. Or consider this list: *calcium, iron, sodium, zinc, thiamin, riboflavin, niacin, ascorbic acid, glucose, sucrose, fructose, xylose, magnesium, nitrate, nitrite, pectin, cellulose, hemicel-*

lulose, lignin, glutamic acid, succinic acid, alpha-ketoglutaric acid, lactic acid, glycolic acid, folic acid, cyanidin 3-(2xylosylgalactoside), cyanidin 3-xylosylglucosylgalactoside, cyanidin 3-ferulylxyloglucosyl galactoside, phenolics, polyacetylenes, and carotenoids. That's an incomplete list of the naturally occurring substances that make up a carrot!

We also know that many of you have questions about supplements, so we include a discussion on how to determine if you might need a supplement and how to choose a supplement if you need one. We believe strongly in a food-first approach, but not necessarily a food-only approach. More information on specific supplements that have evidence to support their use in specific situations is found in Chapter 10. Let's assess your current intake of nutrient-rich foods and supplements:

ASSESS YOURSELF: IN REVIEW

Take the Assess Yourself quiz on the next page before continuing.

We focused first on fruits and vegetables in this assessment because they are so rich in vitamins, minerals, and phytonutrients. You've probably heard about the US Department of Agriculture's 5 A Day for Better Health Program to encourage eating five servings of fruits and vegetables a day, but did you know that five servings is the floor, not the ceiling? Ideally, the goal is to eat nine servings each day! And do you know what is considered as a serving? The good news is that older adults eat more fruits and vegetables than younger age groups, but the bad news is that neither group meets the recommended daily amounts of fruits and vegetables. A worthy goal is to simply eat a little more fruits and vegetables than you currently eat to boost your intake of many essential vitamins, minerals, and phytonutrients. MyPlate also offers daily recommendations for fruits and vegetables (and other food groups) for various age groups. Over age 50, men should be eating about 2½ cups per day of vegetables and 2 cups per day of fruit. These amounts are slightly less for women; 2 cups per day of vegetables and 1½ cups per day of fruit. The table on page 96 and the table on page 97 provide some additional guidance on weekly vegetable subgroup amounts and what is considered a serving of different forms of fruit.

Assess Yourself: Vitamins, Minerals, and Supplements

Do you have a clear picture in your mind of what counts as a serving when you hear "eat at least five servings of fruits and vegetables each day?"

☐ Yes
☐ No

Do you believe that you meet your daily recommended amounts of fruits and vegetables?

☐ Yes
☐ No

Do you know what nutrients are most likely to be in short supply in the diets of those over the age of 50?

☐ Yes
☐ No
☐ Not sure

If yes, which ones?

____

Do you know which vitamins and minerals we need more of as we age? Are there any that we need less of?

☐ Yes
☐ No
☐ Not sure

If yes, which ones?

____

Have you ever had your bone density measured?

☐ Yes
☐ No

If yes, did your doctor tell you that you have low bone mineral density (osteopenia) or that you are at an increased risk for bone fracture (osteoporosis)?

____

Do you think you have an adequate intake of vitamins and minerals from the foods you eat?

☐ Yes
☐ No
☐ Not sure

Have you ever had your vitamin D blood level measured?

☐ Yes
☐ No

If yes, did you doctor tell you that your blood level of vitamin D was low?

____

Do you take vitamin C or other so-called immune-strengthening supplements at the first sign of a cold?

☐ Yes
☐ No

Do you take any vitamin or mineral supplements?

☐ Yes
☐ No

If yes, answer the questions below:

What supplements do you take?

____

How often do you take the supplements, and in what doses?

____

How do you choose a supplement (for example, advice of friends or family, in-store advertising, internet or television advertising, doctor's recommendation)?

____

Do you think natural vitamins are better than synthetic vitamins?

____

Do you take any other type of dietary supplement (herbs, homeopathic, joint health supplements, weight loss, etc)?

____

We'll address your answers to the remaining questions about recommended intakes of vitamins, minerals, and phytonutrients, as well as the potential need for supplements later in this chapter.

TARGET WEEKLY VEGETABLE AMOUNTS FOR MEN AND WOMEN OVER AGE 50

Type of Vegetable	Examples	Amount per Week
Dark green vegetables	Broccoli Greens (collards, mustard, turnips, etc) Kale Raw leafy greens (romaine lettuce, endive, escarole, arugula) Spinach	Men and women: 1½ cups raw or cooked
Red and orange vegetables	Carrots Pumpkin Red peppers Tomato or tomato juice Sweet potato Winter squash	Men: 5½ cups raw or cooked Women: 4 cups raw or cooked
Legumes (also known as pulses)	Beans Lentils Peas	Men: 1½ cups cooked Women: 1 cup cooked
Starchy vegetables	Corn Green peas Potatoes	Men: 5 cups cooked Women: 4 cups cooked
Other vegetables	Bean sprouts Beets Brussels sprouts Cabbage Cauliflower Celery Cucumber Green beans Green peppers Iceberg lettuce Mushrooms Onions Summer squash Zucchini	Men: 4 cups raw or cooked Women: 3½ cups raw or cooked

Adapted from "All About the Vegetable Group," MyPlate, US Department of Agriculture. www.choosemyplate.gov/vegetables.

GUIDE TO UNDERSTANDING FRUIT GROUP SERVINGS

Fruit	What Counts as a 1-cup Serving?
Apple	1 small, ½ large, or 1 cup sliced raw or cooked
Applesauce	1 cup
Banana	1 large
Blueberries, blackberries, raspberries	1 cup
Cantaloupe or honeydew melon	1 cup or ¼ small melon
Grapes	1 cup or 32 seedless
Grapefruit	1 medium or 1 cup sections
Mixed fruit	1 cup (diced or sliced, raw or canned, drained)
Orange	1 large
Orange, mandarin	2 small or 1 cup canned, drained
Peach	1 large or 2 canned halves
Pear	1 medium
Pineapple	1 cup
Plum	3 medium or 2 large
Strawberries	1 cup or 8 large
Watermelon	1 cup or 1-inch-thick slice of small melon
Dried fruit	½ cup
100% fruit juice	1 cup

Adapted from "All About the Fruit Group," MyPlate, US Department of Agriculture.

Knowing if you are getting all of the needed vitamins and minerals can be a challenge. No single blood test can tell if you are getting enough vitamin C or zinc, for example. That's because many vitamins and minerals are part of complex enzyme systems that can't be measured easily (or cheaply!). Even when there is a test to measure blood levels, the experts don't always agree on what constitutes a healthy level.

A case in point is vitamin D: both what is measured and how the measurement is interpreted are debated. Measuring the active form of vitamin D—called 25(OH)D in scientific literature—is the preferred measure, as this form represents both the vitamin D made in your skin from sun exposure as well as vitamin D from food and supplements. If your doctor recommends a blood test, ask about the type of test being performed; how to interpret the results; what it means for you; and whether the results of test indicate that that you should be taking a supplement, and, if so, at what dose.

Keep in mind that knowledge about vitamin D is still emerging, so it isn't surprising that scientists continue to try to pinpoint the healthiest levels of intake for it and the best treatment for deficiencies. It reminds us of measures of cholesterol; in the 1970s, a blood cholesterol of 240 milligrams was considered healthy. Now a blood value of < 200 milligrams is recommended.

In the Assess Yourself box on page 95, we asked about dietary supplements because it is helpful to know what you take, how much you take, and when you take supplements. By doing an inventory of what you take, you might learn that some supplements are duplicative (a multivitamin may contain 100% of the RDA for vitamin C, so there's no need for an additional vitamin C pill) or that you are getting more than the UL for a nutrient. For example, calcium is best absorbed in doses below 500 milligrams. If you take 1,000 milligrams of calcium three times a day, you are over the UL of 2,500 milligrams; plus, a 1,000-milligram dose is not as efficiently absorbed as a 500-milligram dose.

The best strategy to ensure you are getting all of the micronutrients is to eat a variety of foods every day. If, like Candace, you have limited food choices, it is never too late to expand your palate and try new foods and flavors. An easy way to do that is to try one new fruit or vegetable every time you shop for groceries or visit a farmer's market. Just one. Conduct your own taste test with the new food, and you might add something to your usual intake and boost your vitamin and mineral intake. Just as young children often need several tries to learn to like new foods, you may need to try different forms or ways to prepare new fruits and vegetables.

Clarifying the Science on Micronutrients

To clarify the science, we group vitamins and minerals into their various functions in the body. This is a simple approach because some nutrients could be considered in more than one category, and these nutrients are not the only ones needed for the function described in the category. For example, we use the term *energy-assisting nutrients* to describe some of the B vitamins, but this list isn't comprehensive or exhaustive. Also, vitamin B-12 is listed as a blood-building nutrient for its important role in making red blood cells, but it has many other functions. We don't want to exhaust you with too much detail on the function of all vitamins and minerals, but we do provide some useful resources at the end of the chapter for those who want more information.

The need for some vitamins and minerals increases with age, and for two minerals—iron and chromium—decreased intake is recommended. The table on page 101 summarizes the increased and decreased needs for micronutrients for those over age 50. The UL is also listed, which can be used as a guide for the upper limit for supplementation. Many over-50 adults have inadequate intakes of some vitamins and minerals. These shortfall nutrients include calcium, vitamin D, fiber, and potassium, according to the 2015 Dietary Guidelines Advisory Committee.

Vitamins and minerals can be foreign to many and confusing to most, in part because dosage recommendations are made using the metric system. Remember that vitamins and minerals are micronutrients; that is, they are needed in very small amounts. Vitamins and minerals are measured in milligrams (abbreviated mg) or micrograms (abbreviated mcg)—in other words, a thousandth of a gram or one millionth of a gram, respectively. Keep in mind that there are roughly 30 grams in just one ounce. To give you an idea of the scale of the numbers, a teaspoon of salt (a small measure), which is a combination of the minerals sodium and chloride, contains 2,300 milligrams of sodium (a big number using a small unit). Women over 50 need 1,200 milligrams of calcium each day; a multivitamin mineral pill might contain 200 milligrams of calcium and a glass of milk has about 300 milligrams of calcium. And for vitamin D, an older measure called International Units (abbreviated IU) is still used, so we included that measure in the table on page 101.

Energy-Assisting Vitamins (B-1, B-2, B-3)

Everyone wants to have the energy to get through an active day. When we talk about energy, we really are talking about calories. Food is broken down in the gastrointestinal tract into smaller elements that are absorbed into the blood and distributed throughout our bodies. Those small elements are used by a variety of organs and tissues in the body to provide energy to power everything that keeps us alive. B vitamins don't produce energy on their own, but they are like keys that unlock or release the energy found in foods. Processing or milling of grains (bread, cereals, rice) results in a decrease of B vitamins, so most refined grains are enriched, which means these B vitamins (and iron) are added back; folic acid, another B vitamin, is also added. If you see the words thiamin mononitrate, niacin, and riboflavin on the ingredient list, don't be afraid. They are the B vitamins that were in the whole grains before they were made into bread, cereal, pasta, or rice. However, whole grains naturally contain these B vitamins, which is one reason why we encourage whole grains instead of refined grains. The table on the opposite page details why we need these vitamins along with common food sources. Most of us get adequate amounts of these vitamins in our diet because they are widespread in a variety of foods.

Immune-Supporting Nutrients (Vitamin A and Zinc)

Many nutrients are important for a strong immune system, but we singled out two for discussion: vitamin A and zinc (see the table on page 102 for a summary). Vitamin A is classified as a fat-soluble vitamin, and that means it will be better absorbed when taken with a meal that contains some fat. Dipping a carrot stick in hummus or ranch dressing actually improves absorption of the vitamin A (beta carotene) found in the carrot because these foods contain some fat. Vitamin A is unique in that it comes in two forms: preformed (found in animal foods) and precursors, called carotenoids (found in deeply colored fruits and vegetables). When you eat foods with carotenoids, the body converts them to the active form of vitamin A. You might recall that vitamin A plays a role in vision, but it is needed by every cell in the body, especially for healthy skin and the mucous membranes that

AGE-RELATED CHANGES IN VITAMIN AND MINERAL NEEDS FOR ADULTS 50 YEARS AND OLDER

Vitamin or Mineral	Age-Related Change	Amount Needed per Day	Tolerable Upper Limit (UL) Level	Reason for Change
Vitamin D	↑	Women and Men 51–70 years: 15 mcg (600 International Units [IU]) Women and Men over 70 years: 20 mcg (800 IU)	100 micrograms (mcg) (4,000 IU per day)	The skin of older adults has a decreased ability to make Vitamin D, so there are lower levels of the vitamin in the blood.
Vitamin B-12	↑*	2.4 mcg	Not determined	10% to 30% of older adults have trouble absorbing B-12 from food due to changes in stomach acid production. Fortified foods or supplements containing B-12 are recommended to meet daily needs.
Calcium	↑	Women 51–70 years: 1,200 milligrams (mg) Men 51–70 years: 1,000 mg Women and men 71 and over: 1,200 mg	2,500 mg per day	Calcium absorption decreases with age, and intake greater than 1,000 milligrams/day may reduce bone loss.
Iron	↓ (women only)	Women and men over 50 years: 8 mg	45 mg per day	The RDA for women over the age of 50 is reduced to account for the ceasing of menstrual periods.
Chromium	↓	Women over 50 years: 20 mcg Men over 50 years: 30 mcg	Not determined	The need for chromium is tied to calorie intake, so lowered calorie intake among older adults means chromium needs decrease accordingly.

*Although the actual requirement for vitamin B-12 does not change, an increase is noted because absorption is reduced as we age, resulting in a need for adequate vitamin B-12 from supplements or fortified foods.

Source for daily nutrient amounts: Dietary Reference Intakes, Institute of Medicine, National Academy of Sciences.

ENERGY-ASSISTING VITAMINS

Nutrient Common Name (Chemical Name)	Why We Need It	Food Sources
Vitamin B-1 (thiamin)	Helps generate energy from food and transmit nerve impulses	Breakfast cereals fortified with thiamin Enriched breads, cereals, rice, and pasta Whole grains Pork Beans
Vitamin B-2 (riboflavin)	Helps generate energy from food Antioxidant function	Dairy foods Eggs Green leafy vegetables Beef Enriched breads and cereals Chicken Almonds Portabella mushrooms Quinoa
Vitamin B-3 (niacin)	Helps generate energy from food Involved in protein metabolism	Milk Eggs Enriched breads and cereal Rice Fish Lean meats Peanuts Poultry

line the inside of your body. Because the skin and mucous membranes are the first line of defense against infection, vitamin A is needed for a strong immune system, too. Vitamin A is one of the shortfall nutrients for those over 50, even though there are many good food sources.

The precursor form—carotenoids—also acts as an antioxidant. Because of its roles in maintaining healthy cells and as an antioxidant, vitamin A has been studied for cancer prevention. When cancer develops, cells lose their normal function and grow at an uncontrolled rate. People who have diets rich in fruits and vegetables have lower rates for some cancers, and vitamin A and carotenoids are thought to contribute to the reduced rate of cancer. However, don't assume that more is better when it comes to vitamin A. Because it is fat soluble, it can be stored, so consuming too much vitamin A from a supplement can be toxic. With the precursor form of carotenoids, however, the body is smart enough not to convert it all to the active form, thus protecting you from toxicity. Your skin may turn orange (especially the palms of the hands and soles of the feet) if you eat a lot of carrots, but it isn't harmful.

Zinc is a mineral that is a part of hundreds of different enzyme systems in the body that help with all kinds of chemical reactions. Some of the more important functions involve immune function and wound healing. Because of its role in immunity, zinc supplements are widely available over the counter to treat the common cold. Zinc has the potential to inhibit rhinovirus (the virus that causes most colds), which sticks to and replicates in the nose and throat. Zinc might also stop the inflammation that contributes to the symptoms of a cold—runny nose and stuffy head. The research results are mixed, but the latest review from the Cochrane Collaboration (a group that reviews many studies on a particular topic) found that when zinc is taken at the first sign of a cold, the length of the illness is reduced by about 1 day. Is this underwhelming news, or is it worth reducing your cold by about 24 hours? The Commonly Asked Questions section in this chapter, on page 120, gives some additional guidance on zinc supplements.

Bone-Building Nutrients (Calcium, Vitamin D, Magnesium, and Vitamin K)

We are focusing on two vitamins and two minerals for bone health, but, in truth, it takes more than 15 nutrients to build and maintain bones. A summary of bone-building nutrients is found in the table on page 106. Bone is not a static tissue; it undergoes constant turnover, called bone remodeling, to deposit calcium into bones and then remove it (called resorption) to keep blood calcium levels normal. When we are young, we are in the bone-building phase of life, reaching peak bone density in our early teens to mid-20s. Achieving peak bone density (the maximum amount of bone that you can make) helps slow bone loss as we age. As we age, we start to lose more bone than we build—a loss that is greater for women than for men. Estrogen—important for bone health—starts to decline at

NUTRIENTS TO SUPPORT IMMUNE FUNCTION

Nutrient Common Name	Chemical Name	Why We Need it	Food Sources
Vitamin A Carotenoids	Retinol and retinyl ester Beta carotene, alpha carotene, and beta cryptoxanthin	Normal cell development Healthy vision and skin Immune function	***Vitamin A*** Dairy foods Eggs Organ meats (liver) Salmon ***Carotenoids*** Dark green vegetables Carrots Broccoli Sweet potatoes Pumpkins Red peppers Tomatoes Winter squash Cantaloupe Mangos Apricots
Zinc	Zinc	Immune function Wound healing Building new proteins	Seafood Oyster Lobster Crab Meat Beef Pork Dark-meat chicken Baked beans

menopause, and women can lose up to 20% of their bone density in the first 5 to 7 years after menopause. The loss slows after that but never fully recovers. While we think of bone health as a women's issue (80% of those with osteoporosis are women), men are also affected, but usually at later ages. The best things you can do for your bones include the following:

- Get adequate calcium and vitamin D in your diet.
- Exercise—weight-bearing exercise, like walking, jogging, and weight training, is especially important.

- Eat plenty of fruits and vegetables for the micronutrients needed for bone health.
- Do not smoke.
- If you drink alcohol, do so in moderation.

The International Osteoporosis Foundation has an online calculator (see the Useful Resources section on page 126) to help evaluate how much calcium from food and supplements gets into your diet each week.

Calcium Supplements

While foods are the best way to get bone-building nutrients, sometimes supplements are needed to help meet the recommendations for calcium. We will discuss supplements in more detail later in this chapter, but here are some pointers specific to calcium supplements.

- Women and men over the age of 50 need 1,200 milligrams of calcium a day; we suggest you use the International Osteoporosis Foundation's online calcium calculator (see the Useful Resources on page 126) to estimate your calcium intake. If you are below the 1,200-milligram intake level, try to increase your intake of calcium-rich foods. If that isn't possible, consider taking a calcium supplement at the lowest dose needed to get you to 1,200 milligrams a day.
- Calcium comes in many forms; calcium carbonate and calcium citrate are the most common. Calcium carbonate contains 40% usable calcium. This means that a 500-milligram pill provides 200 milligrams of calcium that can be used by the body. Calcium citrate contains 21% usable calcium. Calcium citrate may have a lower amount of usable calcium, but it is better absorbed by older adults than calcium carbonate.
- Calcium is best absorbed in smaller doses, so when taking supplements, don't take more than 500 milligrams of calcium at one time.
- More calcium isn't better: the upper limit is 2,500 milligrams a day, so don't exceed that amount.

BONE-BUILDING NUTRIENTS

Nutrient Common Name	Chemical Name	Why We Need It	Food Sources
Calcium	Calcium	Structure of bones and teeth Transmit nerve signals Cell signals Dilates and contracts blood vessels Muscle function	Dairy foods (milk, cheese, yogurt, cottage cheese, kefir) Fortified milk substitutes (soy, rice, almond, cashew) Sardines Canned salmon Tofu (calcium-set) Turnip greens Kale Almonds Calcium-fortified orange juice Fortified breakfast cereals
Vitamin D	Calcitriol	Promotes calcium absorption from the gut Bone growth and remodeling Regulates cell growth	Fatty fish (salmon, tuna, mackerel, swordfish) Cod liver oil Beef liver Egg yolks Vitamin D–fortified milk, yogurt, orange juice, margarine, breakfast cereals
Magnesium	Magnesium	Bone structure Regulates hundreds of body processes through its role in enzyme systems Regulates blood pressure, blood sugar, and nerve and muscle function	Nuts (almonds, cashews, peanuts) Black beans Edamame Peanut butter Avocado Whole wheat bread Brown rice Potatoes Dairy foods Spinach
Vitamin K	Phylloquinone	Bone metabolism Proteins involved in blood clotting	Leafy green vegetables Spinach Broccoli Soybean and canola oils

Blood-Building Nutrients (Iron, Vitamin B-12, Folic Acid)

We include two water-soluble B vitamins and one mineral as blood-building nutrients, although their importance to health is not limited to making healthy red blood cells. Deficiencies of any of these nutrients result in anemia, which means there are not enough red blood cells in the body or the blood cells are deformed and cannot carry oxygen to tissues.

The most common anemia, iron-deficiency anemia, is probably most familiar. A lack of iron leads to decreasing level of hemoglobin, the oxygen-carrying protein in red blood cells. If you have ever donated blood, you probably had a quick blood test to measure hemoglobin and hematocrit (the percentage of red blood cells in the blood) to make sure you can give blood. With iron-deficiency anemia, both of these measures will be abnormal. Anemia occurs in stages, however, and some people have iron depletion but still have a normal hemoglobin and hematocrit. Symptoms of iron deficiency include excessive tiredness, shortness of breath on simple tasks of exertion, and being cold most of the time. However, don't diagnose yourself with anemia if you have these symptoms; you could be sleep deprived, out of shape, or living in a very cold climate! Another sign of iron-deficiency anemia is something called pica, which is a craving for eating a nonfood item. For example, some pregnant women with severe anemia crave laundry starch or dirt, but a more common craving is to chew crushed or cubed ice. We don't know why this happens, as these substances are not iron rich, but pica is a possible sign of iron-deficiency anemia.

For older adults, iron is still an important nutrient, but women need less iron. After menopause, a woman's need for iron drops to slightly less than half of what it was when she was younger (from 18 milligrams to 8 milligrams.) For men, the need remains at 8 milligrams a day throughout adulthood. Dietary iron comes in two forms: heme iron and nonheme iron. Heme iron (heme means blood) is found in animal-based foods and is better absorbed than the iron found in plant-based foods (nonheme iron). Vegetarians need not worry about getting enough iron; mixing nonheme iron foods with vitamin C enhances absorption. A glass of orange juice with an iron-fortified breakfast cereal, tomato salsa on a bean burrito, and steamed broccoli with a soy veggie burger are good choices to increase the absorption of iron from plants.

Folic acid and vitamin B-12 are needed to help red blood cells mature. A deficiency of these vitamins results in a disorder called megaloblastic anemia ("mega" refers to the big, immature cells). Our need for folic acid and vitamin B-12 remains the same as we age, but a synthetic form of vitamin B-12 is better absorbed than the natural or food form. Since vitamin B-12 is tightly bound to animal-based foods (including dairy and eggs), acid in the stomach is needed to

BLOOD-BUILDING NUTRIENTS

Nutrient Common Name	Chemical Name	Why We Need It	Food Sources
Vitamin B-12	Cobalamin	Makes red blood cells Healthy nerve function Synthesizes DNA	Fish Meat Poultry Eggs Milk Fortified breakfast cereals Some nutritional yeasts
Folate (food form) **Folic acid (fortification and supplement form)**	Folate Folic acid	Synthesizes DNA and RNA Needed for proper cell division Used in protein metabolism	Dark leafy greens Fruit and fruit juice Nuts Beans and peas Dairy foods Asparagus Brussels sprouts Liver
Iron	Iron	Part of hemoglobin in red blood cells and myoglobin in muscles that provides oxygen tissues Part of normal cell function	***Heme and nonheme iron*** Meat Seafood Poultry ***Nonheme iron*** Nuts Beans Iron-fortified grains

free it from the food. Because aging is accompanied by a decrease in stomach acid, the benefit of the synthetic form is that it does not require normal stomach acid for absorption. Vitamin B-12 deficiency can also result in neurologic problems, which is why doctors sometimes check vitamin B-12 levels when an older adult suddenly shows signs of confusion.

If you think you have anemia, don't self-diagnose and devise your own supplement regimen with iron, folic acid, or vitamin B-12. Iron is a prooxidant (more on oxidation in the next section), so more isn't better and, in fact, could be harmful. The same is true of excess folic acid, which could cover up a vitamin B-12 deficiency and cause more harm than good. The best way to get these important nutrients is with food or with a multivitamin and mineral supplement that provides about 100% of the RDA. Blood tests can determine if you have a deficiency, and a doctor can prescribe supplements to treat it. A registered dietitian nutritionist can develop a meal plan to boost these important nutrients if you have a deficiency.

Antioxidant Nutrients (Vitamins C and E)

Part of normal, everyday metabolism produces molecules called free radicals. During aerobic exercise, when you breathe in more oxygen to power working muscles, more free radicals are also produced. These molecules are very unstable and can cause oxidation—modification or destruction of important cell molecules—if they're not neutralized. Don't panic, because oxidation is a normal process, and you see examples of it around you all the time. A car rusting is oxidation, and a fresh avocado slice that turns brown is also oxidation in action. To prevent oxidation, an antioxidant is needed. That is why dipping apple slices in orange juice or squirting lime juice on guacamole prevents browning (the result of oxidation) because the vitamin C in the juice functions as an antioxidant. The table on page 110 provides more details on antioxidant nutrients.

In the body, oxidation can damage cell membranes and structures within the cells, including fats, proteins, and DNA. This damage can set the stage for diseases such as heart disease, some cancers,

COMMON ANTIOXIDANT NUTRIENTS

Nutrients: Common Name	Chemical Name	Why We Need It	Food Sources
Vitamin C	Ascorbic acid	Antioxidant Important in making collagen Needed for wound healing Helps absorb nonheme iron from foods Helps make some neurotransmitters	Red and green peppers Kiwi fruit Oranges and orange juice Grapefruits and grapefruit juice Tangerines Strawberries Broccoli Tomatoes and tomato juice Cantaloupe Cabbage Cauliflower Brussels sprouts
Vitamin E	Alpha-tocopherol	Antioxidant Immune function	Wheat germ Almonds and almond butter Hazelnuts Peanuts and peanut butter Sunflower seeds and oil Safflower oil Corn oil Soybeans and soybean oil Spinach Broccoli
Selenium	Selenium	Antioxidant Immune function Thyroid hormone production	Seafood Organ meats Eggs Grains Brazil nuts

cataract formation, arthritis, and brain and nerve diseases, such as Parkinson's and Alzheimer's. Oxidation is also thought to contribute to accelerating senescence by shortening the ends of chromosomes that direct cell replication and repair. The structures on the ends of chromosomes are called telomeres (think of telomeres as aglets, the plastic coverings at the end of shoelaces). Telomeres shorten as we age, and oxidation can speed up that process. Just like aglets prevent shoelaces from unraveling, antioxidants can help repair damage to shortened telomeres. Before you ask if you should load up on antioxidant supplements to prevent aging, remember that our bodies have several antioxidant defense systems to repair oxidation damage. Some researchers believe that high doses of supplemental antioxidants may actually impair muscle function or delay the training adaptation of muscle. The free radicals might actually have a purpose: signaling the muscle to help it adapt to hard training. For now, the best advice is to avoid taking high-dose supplements and instead eat a wide variety of antioxidant-rich foods. Antioxidants are found not only in fruits and vegetables but also in whole grains, nuts, and seeds.

Phytonutrients

Phytonutrients number in the thousands. Fruits and vegetables contain as many as 20,000 different phytonutrients. The most common and largest group of phytonutrients are called flavonoids, and, to date, more than 4,000 varieties of flavonoids have been identified. Flavonoids share a common chemical structure and are divided into six subclasses, as shown in the table on page 112. One reason why we recommend eating fruits and vegetables instead of relying on supplements is to get the best possible mix of different phytonutrients.

Phytonutrients are thought to be the plant's defense system, protecting it from sun damage, pests, and disease. When humans eat plants, their defense systems come along for the ride, conferring health benefits on the consumer. While researchers are still learning all of the ways plant chemicals work at the cellular level, large-scale studies show that people who eat a lot of phytonutrient-rich foods, beverages, or spices have lower incidences of heart disease, type 2 diabetes, and cancer than those who eat less of them. Phytonutrients are not limited to fruits and vegetables; they are also found in whole grains, pulses, nuts, tea, and some spices. While some powdered extracts and supplements advertised on television and the internet claim that they provide more health benefits than fruits and vegetables, no solid research supports those claims.

PHYTONUTRIENTS

Phytonutrient	Food Sources
Anthocyanidins	Berries Cherries Eggplant Red onions Red potatoes
Flavan-3-ols, flavanols	Dark chocolate Natural cocoa powder Black and green teas Cherries
Flavonols	Apples Kale Leeks Onions
Flavanones	Citrus fruits and juices (orange, grapefruit, lemon)
Flavones	Celery Cherries Parsley Strawberries
Isoflavones	Soybeans Soy flour Soy milk
Lycopene	Tomatoes and tomato products Watermelon Red peppers
Lutein	Dark green leafy vegetables (collard greens, kale, spinach) Broccoli Brussels sprouts Egg yolks Avocados
Resveratrol	Red wine Red grapes Peanuts
Sulforaphanes	Broccoli Brussels sprouts Cabbage Cauliflower
Allicin	Garlic Leeks Shallots Scallions (green onions)

Howard has never met an infomercial he didn't like. He is fascinated with the claims for antiaging supplements that he sees on television. His daily supplement regimen doesn't fit into a standard weekly pillbox that many people use to organize their medicines. He has a tray on his kitchen table to hold the 17 different dietary supplements he takes daily. At 72, Howard says he has never felt better, and he is sure supplements are the secret to healthy aging. As an example, he mentions that the antiarthritis supplements he takes have cured his aching joints. He was a runner until nagging knee and hip pain caused him to stop, but since taking his supplements, he walks several miles each day and has taken up yoga. Howard spends more money on his dietary supplements each month than he does on his Medicare supplemental health insurance. Howard is an example of someone who engages in healthy lifestyle behaviors and is interested in doing everything he can to stay healthy. Unfortunately, many dietary supplements that claim to prevent aging are playing on people's fears of getting older. Some of the supplements in Howard's regimen might be beneficial, but it is unlikely that he needs 17 supplements, at great expense, to get and stay healthy.

Dietary Supplements

Sixty-eight percent of Americans take dietary supplements. A 2015 consumer survey conducted by the Council for Responsible Medicine (an industry trade group representing dietary supplements, ingredient suppliers, and functional food manufacturers) reports that among those age 55 years and older:

- 71% of supplement users take a multivitamin
- 43% of supplement users take vitamin D
- 35% of supplement users take calcium
- 26% of supplement users take vitamin C
- 22% of supplement users take omega-3 fatty acids

The reasons for supplement use in the over-50 group include the following:

- overall health and wellness
- heart health
- bone health
- healthy aging
- fill nutrient gaps in the diet
- maintain healthy cholesterol

For many of us, there are good reasons to take supplements, and supplement users often have healthier habits overall. They tend to eat better, tend to get more exercise, and are more likely to be nonsmokers than nonusers.

What Is a Dietary Supplement?

Dietary supplements are products intended to add nutritional value to our dietary intake. They can include:

- vitamins, such as vitamin C or vitamin B-12
- minerals, such as calcium or magnesium
- herbs or botanicals, such as echinacea or st. john's wort
- amino acids, such as glutamate or branched-chain amino acids
- dietary substances, such as glucosamine and chondroitin or enzymes
- concentrates or extracts, such as green tea or resveratrol

Dietary supplements are regulated by the US Food and Drug Administration (FDA), but they are not as well-regulated as some would like. Those who make and sell dietary supplements are not required to prove that the supplements are pure or safe, or that they work, before bringing them to market. In contrast, drugs and food additives go through a rigorous process before reaching the grocery store or pharmacy shelf. Supplement makers can make claims about the structure or function of a supplement but cannot make a claim about reducing risk of a specific condition or disease. For example, a structure or function claim stating that a suppliment "supports bone health" is allowed, but it might be interpreted as "builds and maintains good bone health and reduces the risk of osteoporosis," even though this specific language is not allowed. In addition, every supplement that carries a structure or function claim on the label must also include this disclaimer: "This statement has not been evaluated by the FDA. This product is not intended to diagnose, treat, cure, or prevent any disease."

Howard is trying hard to stay healthy, and we applaud him for that. Howard is not unusual in believing his supplements have cured his arthritis. Those who have arthritis know it is a fickle disease; some days are worse than others. A supplement taken on Monday or Tuesday may be credited for its healing powers if the person's arthritis is not painful on Wednesday or Thursday. Howard did other things that might have helped his arthritis: he gave up running and taking up yoga. Both of those changes could have helped his arthritic knee pain. Glucosamine and chondroitin supplements may provide some benefit to arthritis joint pain, but they aren't a miracle cure, nor do those supplements work for everyone. We would suggest that Howard review all of his supplements and look beyond the manufacturer's claims. Unfortunately, the marketing is often ahead of the science when it comes to claims of potential benefits for supplements. Resources to evaluate supplements are found at the end of the chapter.

How Do You Know If You Need Dietary Supplements?

Knowing what supplements might be beneficial requires knowing what nutrients you get in your diet. If you don't eat fatty fish, such as salmon or herring, you might consider taking a fish oil or omega-3 fatty acid supplement. Ask yourself these questions before taking supplements:

- Is my diet all that it could be in terms of eating a variety of healthy foods, including at least five servings of fruits and vegetables each day?
- Am I consuming enough calories (energy) every day to support my activity? Chronic dieting and focusing only on calories for weight loss can lead to restrictive food choices.

- Am I choosing whole grains or enriched grains to make sure I am getting enough B vitamins from my diet?
- Am I eating protein-rich foods throughout the day? Protein-rich foods are often the best source of minerals in our diet.
- If I don't eat meat, am I getting protein substitutes, like soy or beans, in my diet?
- What specifically do I want to accomplish by using dietary supplements?
- Am I getting unbiased information on supplements, or do I just rely on the supplement maker's claims or information I read on the internet or hear from friends or family members?
- If someone is trying to persuade you to take supplements, does this person have a vested interest in selling supplements (eg, a financial incentive or multilevel marketing system that accrues benefits for the seller)?

We encourage you to ask your doctor or qualified health professional (like a registered dietitian nutritionist) about what supplements might be beneficial for you, and do some investigating on your own using the resources found at the end of the chapter.

How to Choose a Dietary Supplement

We think it is important to get information on supplements from a credible source. Anecdotes from other supplement users should not be the only reason to take a supplement. Use some of the resources listed at the end of this chapter for an objective evaluation of supplements. If your research is limited to an internet search on a supplement, you are likely to get advertisements from those trying to sell the supplement or testimonials from those who have a vested interest in getting you to buy it.

Once you decide on a supplement, look for third-party verification that you are getting a quality supplement. Have you ever noticed the USP symbol on a supplement? That stands for United States Pharmacopeia, and it means the supplement meets strict voluntary criteria for quality ingredients and quality manufacturing processes. ConsumerLab.com is another group that tests supplements to make sure the supplement contains what the label says it does. Third-party verification doesn't mean the product will work for you, but it does ensure that you are getting what you are paying for.

Take supplements according to the dosing instructions, and make sure to check sources such as the National Institute of Health Office of Dietary Supplements for drug–supplement interactions. For example, St. John's wort activates enzymes in the liver, which in turn reduces the concentration of some drugs in the blood, such as digoxin, a drug used to treat congestive heart failure.

Remember that supplements are a *supplement* to your diet—eating poorly and expecting a supplement to keep you healthy is wishful thinking. Also, some supplements take time to work; they are not like antibiotics that can cure an infection in a couple of days. For example, glucosamine and chondroitin may help some with osteoarthritis, but it can take months to know if the supplement is working. Lastly, if claims for supplements sound too good to be true, then they probably are. Think about how many people say that vitamin C is the cure for the common cold. If that were true, wouldn't everyone take vitamin C and never suffer through another cold again? So, be realistic about your expectations for supplements.

Confronting the Myths About Vitamins, Minerals, and Phytonutrients

MYTH: Canned or frozen foods contain no vitamins or minerals.

REALITY: Bashing processed foods is popular today, but commercially canned or frozen vegetables and fruits can actually have more vitamins or minerals than fresh foods, depending on when the fresh food was picked, how it was transported, and how long it remained in storage. A study from the University of California–Davis evaluated eight common fresh fruits and vegetables compared with the same frozen foods and found that the nutrient values were the same, and in some cases higher, than in the fresh foods. Foods destined for canning or freezing are picked at the peak of ripeness and transported to processing facilities, often a short distance from the field, where they are quickly canned or frozen. Freezing and canning also extends the time that we can enjoy out-of-season produce and boost our nutrient intake, and these foods don't require preservatives because the processing acts to preserve the food. Some canned vegetables do contain added sodium, but not all do. Sure, nothing beats a fresh-picked tomato from your garden for taste and nutrition, but we all don't have the ability or time to grow our own food year-round, so don't worry about eating frozen and canned produce to round out your garden's bounty.

MYTH: Microwaving destroys nutrients.

REALITY: Overcooking can destroy nutrients, especially the water-soluble B vitamins and vitamin C, but microwaving actually helps preserve nutrients because of the short cooking time. Microwaving, steaming, and roasting all preserve nutrients. If you boil your veggies, you will lose some of the vitamins to the cooking water, but save the liquid and use it in soups or stews for a vitamin-enriched broth.

MYTH: Raw foods are best.

REALITY: Raw foods can be healthy, but we wouldn't say they are the best. Cooking helps make some nutrients more available to be absorbed. Lycopene, the phytonutrient that gives tomatoes their red color, is better absorbed when cooked; it has up to 55% greater absorption ability than when eaten raw. Canned tomatoes, tomato sauce, tomato soup, marinara sauce, and ketchup are all examples of cooked tomato products that deliver more lycopene than raw tomatoes. Other vegetables, such as kale, carrots, spinach, mushrooms, asparagus, cabbage, and peppers, also deliver more nutrients when cooked versus raw. And we know that consuming raw foods, such as sprouts, raw milk, and raw-milk cheeses and yogurt, increases the risk of food poisoning.

MYTH: Vitamin A will improve my vision.

REALITY: Vitamin A is an important part of the visual cycle; its chemical name, retinol, indicates its role in helping light get to the retina of the eye. Vitamin A deficiency can lead to blindness, and in developing countries, this is a major problem. However, the common vision-related change as we age, farsightedness requiring bifocals, is not related to vitamin A intake.

MYTH: B vitamins improve your energy level.

REALITY: It is easy to see why B vitamins are equated with energy, as their role inside our cells is to help unlock the energy stored in food. But by themselves, they do not make us feel energized. In nutrition, energy is another word for calories. If energy bars were called calorie bars, we think no one but the most avid exerciser would eat them.

MYTH: Avoid enriched or fortified foods and eat only natural foods.

REALITY: Let's take a minute to understand these terms. We've mentioned enrichment in the section on B vitamins. *Enrichment* is the addition of a nutrient that was lost in processing. Enriched grains, for example, contain the B vitamins thiamin, riboflavin, and niacin, as well as the mineral iron. *Fortification* is the addition of a nutrient to a food that doesn't naturally contain significant amounts of the vitamin or mineral. Fortification of the food supply began as a public health measure. For example, the mineral iodine is added to salt to prevent a thyroid condition called goiter caused by iodine deficiency. Vitamin D is added to milk to help us absorb calcium. Without vitamin D, only 10% to 15% of calcium is absorbed. Folic acid fortification is required in refined grains to reduce the incidence of birth defects of the spine and brain (and since this fortification program was introduced in 1998, the number of babies born with spine and brain defects has decreased 25% to 30%). So there is good reason to enrich or fortify some foods with some nutrients, but not always. For example, adding vitamin C to a sugary drink doesn't turn it into a healthy food.

MYTH: Chromium supplements prevent diabetes.

REALITY: Chromium is an important cofactor in controlling blood sugar and, thus, is sometimes called the "glucose tolerance factor." However, supplemental chromium will not prevent or treat diabetes. Chromium is a trace mineral, meaning it is needed in very small amounts. Food sources include broccoli, potatoes, meat and poultry, and some herbs, like basil.

Commonly Asked Questions About Vitamins, Minerals, and Phytonutrients

Do zinc supplements prevent the common cold?

As we discussed earlier in the chapter, zinc might have some modest effect on reducing cold symptoms. Here are some things to consider if you want to try zinc lozenges:

- Timing and dose are important; try one zinc lozenge at the first sign of a cold, and repeat every 4 hours.
- More isn't better; in fact, it can make things worse; nausea and vomiting can occur with high doses of zinc, and it can leave a metallic taste in your mouth.
- High doses of zinc supplements can interfere with absorption of other minerals needed for good health.
- Avoid zinc nasal sprays. The Food and Drug Administration warned consumers that zinc sprays can lead to sometimes permanent changes in the sense of smell.
- Zinc can interfere with some prescription medications, such as antibiotics and blood thinners, so always consider potential drug interactions

Do calcium supplements cause heart attacks in women who take supplements?

Calcium from your diet or supplements does not contribute to heart attacks. When the inside lining of the arteries that carry blood to the heart (coronary arteries) are damaged or injured by high blood pressure, high blood lipids, or the chemicals in cigarette smoke, inflammation takes place. Calcium is deposited in the artery as a response to the injury, as it is a major player in scar formation, but calcium doesn't cause heart disease. Aim to meet your daily requirements for calcium with food and/or supplements; more isn't better, however, as is true for any vitamin or mineral.

If my blood calcium level is in the normal range, does that mean my bone density is also normal?

Blood calcium represents a tiny fraction of the total calcium in the body—only about 1%. That small amount is critical to keeping our hearts beating and transmitting signals from the nervous system to help control hundreds of body functions. When blood levels of calcium fall too low, calcium is released from bone to keep things normal. That is why your bone density test, not your blood level of calcium, is the best measure to know if your bones are strong.

What is the difference between vitamin D-2 and D-3 in supplements? Is one form preferred over another?

Two forms of vitamin D are used in supplements and fortified foods: D-2 (called ergocalciferol) and D-3 (called cholecalciferol). While both forms can help raise vitamin-D blood levels, the D-3 form has the edge over D-2 for more potency.

Do proton pump inhibitor drugs taken to treat gastric reflux cause vitamin deficiencies?

Drugs used to treat gastric reflux and ulcer disease work by slowing the release of stomach acid. Vitamin B-12 from food needs stomach acid for proper digestion and absorption, so theoretically these drugs could reduce the availability of this vitamin. However, there is not a lot of evidence to suggest that they cause a vitamin deficiency. Still, long-term users should talk to their doctors and ask to have vitamin B-12 levels monitored. Vitamin B-12 from supplements is readily absorbed without stomach acid, so ask your doctor if a supplement is needed.

Having the Confidence to Make Food Choices that Provide Vitamins, Minerals, and Phytonutrients

One assignment that we used when teaching nutrition was the dreaded 3-day food dairy, where students were required to analyze their usual diet for vitamin and mineral intake. Although students dreaded the tedious nature of logging everything they ate and drank, they often said it was the most useful assignment they ever completed to learn about nutrients. If taking stock of your nutrient intake is something that interests you, there are some easy and free tools to help you do just that, such as Super Tracker, which can be done on your computer, tablet, or smartphone (see the Useful Resources section on page 125). Using a tracker would help Candice see that while her diet has enough calories and carbohydrate, she is woefully short of many vitamins and minerals. A tracker can show her where she could add a food or two to boost nutrient intake. Sometimes adding just one serving of a food can have a big impact on improving intake. For example, if Candice added an 8-ounce glass of calcium-fortified 100% orange juice, she could get about one-third of her daily calcium needs, 25% of vitamin D, 15% of folic acid, and 100% of vitamin C for just 110 calories.

Increasing vitamins, mineral, and phytonutrients at every meal is actually quite easy. Look for ways to add fruits and veggies or nuts and seeds into your usual meals. For years, the term *stealth health* was used to describe the practice of sneaking fruits and veggies into dishes to disguise them. But most older adults know the value of including more fruits and veggies in their diet and don't have to resort to the sneaky approach. Try to add a serving of fruit or veggies to every meal to easily push the number of servings upward. Every extra serving helps. The box on the oppoiste page has a few suggestions to get you started.

Conversation with an Expert

Scott Powers, PhD, a Distinguished Professor and the UAA Endowed Professor at the University of Florida, is known for his expertise in antioxidants and exercise. He describes his background as follows:

> My interest in exercise-induced radical production began in the late 1980s. At that time, exercise-induced radical production was viewed as an "unwanted" consequence of muscular exercise. Indeed, because exercise was

INCREASING VITAMINS, MINERALS, AND PHYTONUTRIENTS

Breakfast

Drink low-fat or nonfat milk or calcium-fortified 100% juice.
Add fresh berries, bananas, or peaches to cereal.
Add black beans to scrambled eggs and top with salsa.
Add dried fruit to oatmeal.
Make smoothies with fresh or unsweetened frozen fruit.
Fold berries into pancake or waffle batter.
Sauté mushrooms, peppers, onions, and broccoli and add to scrambled eggs or an omelet.
Top frozen waffles with fresh or frozen strawberries instead of syrup.

Lunch

Make a wrap with cheese or turkey, chopped tomatoes, and leftover salad.
Substitute carrots, celery, cucumbers, or other crunchy veggies for chips.
Add banana pepper rings to sandwiches.
Choose a veggie sandwich over a meat-filled one.
Add mixed fruit and chopped nuts to vanilla Greek yogurt.
Add thinly sliced apple or pear to a sandwich.
Choose tomato-based soups or gazpacho instead of cream soups.
Drain a can of vegetables, and then add it to a pot of broth-based soup.
Add avocado slices to sandwiches and salads.

Dinner

When eating pizza, whether take-out or homemade, choose more veggie toppings than meat toppings, and go easy on the cheese.
Roast cherry tomatoes in the oven with a drizzle of olive oil and serve over hot pasta.
Switch to dark, leafy greens for salads instead of just iceberg lettuce.
Add drained and rinsed canned chickpeas or other legumes to salads.
Learn to roast vegetables for rich flavors; try roasting cauliflower, broccoli, Brussels sprouts, onions, asparagus, turnips, and sweet potatoes with a drizzle of olive oil in the oven or on the grill.
Sauté green peas and bean sprouts with leftover rice for a quick fried rice.
Blend chopped mushrooms into lean ground beef or turkey for juicy, vegetable-rich burgers, taco meat, or meatloaf.
Try fruit-based desserts for a sweet ending; bake apples or pears and top with oatmeal crumble and vanilla yogurt.

Snacks

Cut up melons and store in covered containers in the fridge for quick snacks.
Keep a fruit bowl on the kitchen counter; if fruit gets overripe, use it in a smoothie.

> associated with oxidative stress, some "experts" recommended that athletes and other physically active people support their diet with antioxidant supplements. Fast-forward 25 years. It is now clear that exercise-induced production of radicals in skeletal muscles plays an important role in promoting muscle adaptation to exercise, and that supplementation with "mega-doses" of antioxidant vitamins (eg, vitamins E and C) can blunt exercise-induced "healthy" adaptations in skeletal muscles.

Now in his mid-60s, Scott enjoys the many health benefits associated with regular exercise and is active 6 or 7 days each week. He describes his eating habits as "three well-balanced and isocaloric [similar calorie amount] meals a day; unfortunately, this goal is not always achieved." In that regard, he is like most of us.

As he ages, he says he doesn't "waste valuable time worrying about the negative aspects of growing older. Instead, I choose to invest my time enjoying intellectual activities (eg, doing research, reading, and writing) and engaging in regular endurance and resistance exercise training. Also, an occasional trip to the ocean is time well spent, and we should all watch as many sunsets over the ocean as possible."

How the Authors Get Vitamins, Minerals, and Phytonutrients

Chris: I like vegetables more than fruit (except for clementine tangerines, which I eat every day in season). I love stir-frying vegetables with small amounts of chicken, shrimp, beef, or tofu. My other favorite way to cook vegetables is roasting them in the oven with a drizzle of flavored olive oil (garlic, lemon, and Tuscan herb-infused olive oils are always in my kitchen). I bring roasted cauliflower and broccoli to family gatherings, where they are eaten with enthusiasm, even by those who say they don't like vegetables. As for supplements, I take a multivitamin/mineral formulated for women over 50; while I eat well, I like the added security of knowing I am getting the trace minerals found in the multivitamin, along with added calcium and vitamin D. I also take omega-3 supplements because I don't eat enough fatty fish.

Bob: I take a daily vitamin D supplement, doubling the dose in the gray winter months, but rely on my diet to supply all the other micronutrients I need. There aren't many foods I don't like, and I enjoy a lot of variety in my diet, including fruits and vegetables. I like to use frozen mixed berries on cereal and in smoothies, along with snacking on whatever fruits and vegetables I find in my refrigerator. My wife has similar dietary habits, and because she does most of the shopping and cooking, I find it easy to eat a varied diet.

Useful Resources

Vitamin, Mineral, and Phytonutrient Resources

American Cancer Society (www.cancer.org/healthy/eathealthygetactive/acsguidelinesonnutritionphysicalactivityforcancerprevention/index?ssSourceSiteId=null)

▷ *ACS Guidelines on Nutrition and Physical Activity for Cancer Prevention is updated about every 5 years to reflect the science on the role of diet and exercise on cancer prevention*

American Institute for Cancer Research (www.aicr.org/foods-that-fight-cancer)

▷ *AICR's Foods that Fight Cancer list is regularly updated as more is learned about the roles of specific foods in cancer prevention.*

Office of Disease Prevention and Health Promotion (http://health.gov/dietaryguidelines)

▷ *Dietary Guidelines for Americans, updated every 5 years, offers a wealth of information on nutrition, food choices, and how the whole family can eat healthy*

Produce for Better Health Foundation, Fruits and Veggies—More Matters (www.fruitsandveggiesmorematters.org)

▷ *Variety of information on the role of fruits and vegetables in promoting good health*

Dietary Supplement Resources

Aegis Shield (www.aegisshield.com)

▷ *Lists of supplements with banned performance-enhancing ingredient;, may be helpful for Master's athletes who compete in sporting events*

ConsumerLab.com (www.consumerlab.com)

▷ *Subscription site that evaluates dietary supplements to ensure they contain what the label says they contain; also provides expert evaluation and frequently asked questions on a variety of supplement topics*

Council for Responsible Nutrition (www.crnusa.org)

▷ *Industry trade group providing consumer education on supplements, statistics on supplement use, information on how to read a supplement label, and fact sheets on various supplements*

International Osteoporosis Foundation (www.iofbonehealth.org/calcium-calculator)

▷ *Online calculator to help evaluate how much calcium from food and supplements gets into your diet each week.*

MyPlate.gov (www.supertracker.usda.gov)

▷ *MyPlate's Supertracker site allows you to create a personalized nutrition and physical activity plan and track foods and physical activities*

National Institutes of Health, Office of Dietary Supplements (https://ods.od.nih.gov)

▷ *Reliable scientific information on vitamins, minerals, and dietary supplements, including functions, daily needs, food sources, and more*

Natural Medicines Comprehensive Database (http://naturaldatabase.therapeuticresearch.com/home.aspx?cs=&s=ND)

▷ *Subscription site; offers detailed scientific research on complementary, alternative, and integrative nutrition*

Nutrition.gov, Dietary Supplements (www.nutrition.gov/dietary-supplements)

▷ *Aggregates many government websites that address dietary supplements*

US Food and Drug Administration (www.fda.gov/Food/DietarySupplements/UsingDietarySupplements/default.htm)

▷ *Information on using dietary supplements, including safety and how to report an adverse reaction to a supplement*

US National Library of Medicine, Medline Plus (www.nlm.nih.gov/medlineplus/druginfo/herb_All.html)

▷ *A-Z listing of dietary supplements and herbal remedies with information on their effectiveness, usual dosage, drug interactions, and more*

SECTION 2

MOVE WELL

THIS SECTION OF the book is devoted to the importance of moving well—and doing so on a daily basis for the rest of our lives. After all, our health, happiness, and overall quality of life—our ability to be well—are directly affected by eating well and moving well.

We can't imagine there are any American adults over the age of 50 who haven't heard that regular physical activity plays an important role in living a long and healthy life. We *can* imagine that most of those 50-plusers would like to be more physically active but are constrained by busy schedules, a disdain for exercise, or an inability to overcome the inertia of many years of relative inactivity. Indeed, a body at rest will remain at rest unless an external force—or internal motivation—determines otherwise.

One famous American who supposedly disdained physical activity was Mark Twain (Samuel Langhorne Clemens). Twain was born in 1835 and died at age 75 in 1910, a respectable life span in those times. It's not entirely clear what Twain's personal habits were when it came to regular exercise, but he certainly contributed some memorable quotes on the subject, including these:

"I'm pushing sixty. That's enough exercise for me."

"I have never taken any exercise, except sleeping and resting, and I never intend to take any."

Twain is often wrongly credited for another famous quote, the author of which is still undetermined: "Whenever I get the urge to exercise, I lie down until the feeling passes." Twain may have never engaged in organized sports or participated in regular exercise, such as jogging or weight lifting, but he was undoubtedly physically active by virtue of the times in which he lived. Walking and horseback riding were common modes of transportation in Twain's times, and, along with the basic chores required for daily living, they provided ample physical activity for most.

But times have certainly changed, and they continue to change, making it easier to lead a sedentary lifestyle today than ever before. In 2016, the Centers for Disease Control and Prevention released a report, "Physical Inactivity Among Adults Aged 50 Years and Older—United States, 2014," in which roughly 28% of those surveyed (more than 275,000 people) reported no physical activity during the most recent month. Inactivity increased with age, and 35% of those over 75 years reported being inactive.

The intent of this section is not to hammer you over the head with statistics about inactivity or dire pronouncements about its health risks but to first and foremost impress upon you that *avoiding inactivity* should be everyone's goal. Some readers might be delighted to learn that avoiding inactivity does not require new exercise clothes or membership to a health club. It simply requires a personal commitment to sitting less and moving more. For some people, the moving more part of the equation might mean walking around the neighborhood instead of watching television, while for others it might mean signing up for a fitness class or dusting off the treadmill in the basement. In essence, moving more means whatever you'd like it to mean, just as long as you are truly moving more for at least 30 minutes each day.

There are plenty of ways to move well, so let's get started.

CHAPTER

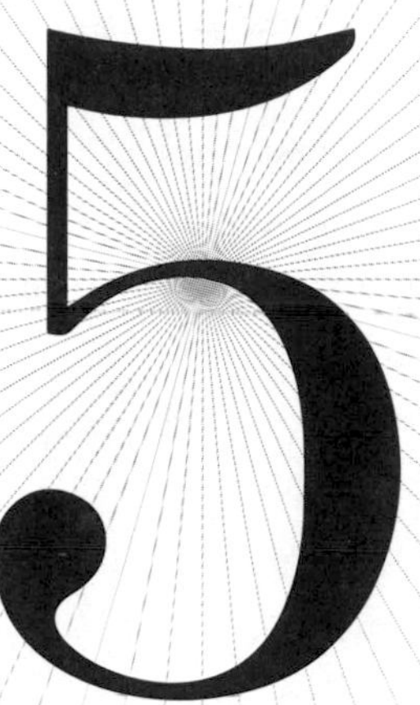

HOW TO GET AND STAY IN SHAPE

The Bottom Line

For most Americans, increasing daily physical activity should be their top health priority because inactivity is the enemy of good health. It's easy to fall into a sedentary rut, where prolonged sitting at work and home is the rule rather than the exception. Our bodies are built to move, to be active, to get things done, and to have fun. The demands of being physically active cause our bodies to adapt and change in ways that make us more capable of meeting future demands. Those adaptations not only improve our fitness but also have enormous benefits for our health—benefits that no prescription drug can match. Here are some key points to keep in mind:

- Physical fitness declines as we age, but we have control over the rate of that decline.
- Staying physically active throughout life may be one of the most important factors in living a long, happy, and healthy life.

- **There are endless ways to be physically active—on your own, with friends, or in exercise classes. If the thought of exercise turns you off, keep in mind that the best activities for our health are the ones we enjoy most because those are the activities we will continue doing.**
- **Take advantage of every opportunity to move; this not only improves health and fitness but also contributes to managing or losing weight by increasing the number of calories burned each day.**

Introduction

In the middle of the night, a few months shy of her 60th birthday, Ruth experienced severe abdominal pain. Friends rushed her to the local emergency department where surgeons repaired an aneurysm in her abdominal aorta, saving her life. Looking back, Ruth realized that she had lost her normal levels of physical and mental energy over the prior year, a change that was so gradual she didn't even notice. Now, with a second chance at life, Ruth plans to make the most of it and knows she has to do a better job of keeping fit. She was a good athlete in high school and college, but she put on 60 extra pounds soon after marriage. After 18 years of being obese (peak weight of 255 pounds on a 5-foot 6-inch body, giving her a body mass index [BMI] of 36.3—in the obese category), Ruth successfully lost 125 pounds and has kept it off for over 10 years, a remarkable success by any measure. Now at 130 pounds, Ruth's BMI is a healthy 21.0. The aneurysm was a major setback but also a stark reminder that Ruth needed to improve her physical capacity if she wanted to continue to live on her own and enjoy life. Her two dogs have made getting out of the house for walks a part of her daily routine, but Ruth realizes that dog walks won't be enough to give her the health and vitality needed to accomplish all the things she'd like. Like many older adults, Ruth wants to become more fit but is not sure where to start or how to progress. She knows that walking more would be a good foundation for whatever additional exercise she decides to pursue and has upped her daily walking distance and pace. Ruth has heard that some health plans for older adults offer no-cost fitness memberships through programs such as Tivity Health's SilverSneakers, a national network of fitness programs. She will also look into joining a local YMCA or fitness club to see if that will fit into her budget and schedule.

To start, we should define physical fitness as "good health, strength, and physical stamina achieved through regular physical activity." But being "fit" or "in shape" means different things to different people. For some, fitness means being able to work hard in training sessions and competitions, while for others, it may mean looking healthy and lean, or simply getting through each day without feeling exhausted. Another term to be aware of is functional fitness—being physically capable of accomplishing your goals and enjoying the health benefits that come along with improved fitness. Our purpose in these next three chapters is to share knowledge and suggestions to help you improve your overall physical and functional fitness.

The Physical Activity Guidelines for Americans, also discussed in Chapter 1, were established to identify the amount and intensity of weekly physical activity that is known to produce health benefits, such as decreased risk of heart disease, heart attacks, diabetes, some cancers, and osteoporosis (low bone density); reduce pain from arthritis; delay onset of Alzheimer's disease and dementia;, and increase life expectancy. The box at the right is a reminder of the physical activity guidelines and also defines moderate and vigorous intensity exercise. Sadly, 90% of American adults do not meet these physical activity guidelines. Despite benefits that no prescription drug or dietary supplement can match, physical activity among American adults continues to decline.

Physical Activity Guidelines for Americans

150 minutes per week of moderate-intensity activity or 75 minutes each week of vigorous-intensity activity

Strength training at least twice each week.

Next, let's distinguish activity that is moderate intensity from vigorous intensity: If you can talk during exercise but not sing an entire song, that's moderate-intensity activity. If you are huffing and puffing and can speak only a few words at a time, that's vigorous-intensity exercise. Low-intensity activity—when you can talk or sing—is still much better for your health than no exercise at all, so take advantage of every opportunity to move. If 75 to 150 minutes of exercise each week seems daunting, don't despair. There is a viable time-saving option—high-intensity interval training—described later in the chapter.

However—and this is an important however—even if we do meet the physical activity guidelines, the health benefits produced by improved fitness can be counteracted by prolonged sitting. Too much sitting is associated with a wide waist, high blood pressure, high blood triglycerides, and low levels of high-density lipoprotein cholesterol, all of which are bad for health. In short, too much sitting increases the risk of cardiovascular disease and early death. If you have to sit a lot, being fit is even more important because fitness protects us from some—but not all—of the risks of prolonged sitting. A good rule of thumb is to do 10 minutes of physical activity for every hour of sitting; research shows that it takes an hour of activity to offset the negative impact of 8 hours of sitting. Happily, we can spread that hour of activity across the day in smaller increments of activity.

If you already meet the weekly guidelines for physical activity, that's fantastic, but remember that being fit doesn't absolve us of other lifestyle sins. As the saying goes, "you can't outrun a bad diet." With that adage in mind, scientists estimate that only 2.7% of American adults satisfy four reasonable criteria for leading a healthy lifestyle: regularly consuming a balanced diet, refraining from smoking, maintaining a body fat percentage in the acceptable range, and meeting the physical activity guidelines. Regardless of our lifestyle choices, any physical activity is better for our health than no physical activity: replacing just 30 minutes of sedentary time with physical activity reduces all-cause mortality (death from all possible health-related causes).

Assess Yourself: Physical Fitness

What would you like your fitness routine to accomplish in the next 6 months?

- ☐ Weight loss
- ☐ Improved health
- ☐ Muscle tone
- ☐ Enhanced sports performance
- ☐ Maintenance of current fitness

What would you like your fitness routine to accomplish as you grow older?

____

How many hours each day do you spend sitting in the following locations:

- ☐ At the table: ____
- ☐ In your car: ____
- ☐ At your desk : ____
- ☐ In front of the television or other screen (computer, phone, or tablet): ____

How many hours each day do you spend sleeping?

- ☐ Less than 6 hours
- ☐ 6 to 8 hours
- ☐ More than 8 hours

Calculate the percent of the day you spend sitting (as a percentage of your waking hours) using the following equation:

$$\frac{\#\text{Sitting Hours}}{\#\text{Standing Hours}} \times 100 = \_\_\_\_\_\_$$

On average, how long do you sit before getting up to move around?

- ☐ 30 minutes or less
- ☐ 30 to 60 minutes
- ☐ 60 to 90 minutes
- ☐ More than 90 minutes

When you do get up and move around, how long do you usually do so?

- ☐ Less than 15 minutes
- ☐ 15 to 45 minutes
- ☐ More than 45 minutes

How much time do you typically spend watching television or at the computer?

- ☐ Less than 1 hour
- ☐ 1 to 3 hours
- ☐ More than 3 hours

What are your four favorite kinds of physical activity?

____

How much time each day do you devote to a formal exercise session (eg, walking, jogging, biking, swimming, resistance training, fitness class, personal trainer)?

- ☐ Less than 20 minutes
- ☐ 20 to 40 minutes
- ☐ 40 to 60 minutes
- ☐ More than 60 minutes

How much time each day would you like to be able to devote to exercise?

- ☐ Less than 20 minutes
- ☐ 20 to 40 minutes
- ☐ 40 to 60 minutes
- ☐ More than 60 minutes

When during the day is the best time for you to exercise?

- ☐ Morning
- ☐ Afternoon
- ☐ Evening

Have you used—or do you currently use—a fitness device to keep track of your daily activity?

- ☐ Yes
- ☐ No

Do you typically meet or exceed your fitness tracking goals?

- ☐ Yes
- ☐ No

ASSESS YOURSELF: IN REVIEW

Take the Assess Yourself quiz on the previous page before reading on.

You might have been shocked by the total amount of time you spend sitting (and sleeping) during a typical day. All those hours are sedentary time involving little to no movement. While getting enough sleep each night is good for health, prolonged sitting is bad, so we should all strive to sit less and break up the periods of time when we do sit. Many jobs require prolonged sitting, and it's understandable that hours can whiz by before we realize that we haven't moved from our workstation. That much sitting is bad news for health and longevity, so if you only adopt one new behavior from this chapter, we hope it's to reduce the time you spend sitting during work and while you are at home. Although that doesn't sound like much of a fitness recommendation, it actually is.

As you'll read in this chapter, regular physical activity—even low-level activity—is more potent than any drug at benefiting your health in a wide assortment of ways, both physical and mental. If you don't currently exercise on a regular basis, try starting by setting aside just 15 minutes of your day to devote to whatever activity interests you. Once you become accustomed to establishing time for regular exercise, it's much easier to increase the intensity and duration of your activity. In other words, it's much easier to modify an existing habit than to create a new one. For those new to exercise, starting slowly and increasing gradually is the best way to improve fitness over the long term. For many of us, finding the time each day to exercise is much more difficult than the exercise itself!

Once you've identified your short-term and long-term fitness goals, you're ready to begin the journey to a healthier you. Before you begin, it's always helpful to seek the advice of your physician along with exercise specialists, such as those at the local YMCA, health club, or college. You might also want to try a personal trainer to help you get started. Qualified exercise specialists are trained to help people design and implement fitness programs tailored to individual needs and interests. Ask about the trainer's credentials and do a little research on the internet to satisfy yourself that the credentials are legitimate. Don't be shy about making clear your goals, interests, and limitations because you have to be 100% satisfied with the plan. It's also important to make sure that you receive periodic feedback along the way so you can get a sense of your progress and fine-tune your fitness program as time goes by. You can do that on your own, perhaps by using a wearable fitness monitor, if you enjoy that kind of feedback, or with the help of a fitness-class instructor or personal trainer.

Aging and Fitness

Hippocrates said something along the lines of this: "Eating alone will not keep a man well; he must also take exercise. For food and exercise...work together to produce health." It's amazing that Hippocrates's advice, given more than 1,500 years ago, has seemingly been all but lost over the intervening millenniums. Of course, it wasn't that long ago that most occupations and lifestyles involved considerable physical activity. This characteristic has changed markedly over just the past few decades—changes that anyone over 50 has witnessed firsthand. Other relatively recent changes are that we eat at restaurants more often and that meal portion sizes in most homes and restaurants are larger than ever before. We'll discuss this more in Chapter 8, which covers weight management.

Consider for a moment the finding that the decrease in housework that has occurred since the 1960s is associated with an increase in body fat—and in the prevalence of overweight and obesity—among American women. Researchers noted that the average woman in the 1960s spent about 25 hours each week doing household chores such as laundry, cleaning, cooking, dishwashing, and vacuuming. (Yes, housework counts as physical activity.) By 2015, that figure was cut in half. Over the same span, the average woman also became more engaged in sedentary activities, including desk work; reading; and screen time spent in front of televisions, smartphones, tablets, and computers. The same trends are true for men. Reduced physical activity—and the drop in energy (calorie) expenditure that goes along with it—has made us collectively fatter and less fit.

We are not going to spend time reviewing all of the age-related changes that affect our physical fitness, so if you are interested in those details, peruse the information in the box below.

Age-Related Changes that Affect Physical Fitness

Many normal changes that occur as we age influence our overall physical fitness and challenge our ability to live happy, healthy, and independent lives. The goal of remaining physically active is to reduce the rate at which the following changes occur.

- Lower maximal heart rate
- Reduced stroke volume (the amount of blood pumped by the heart with each beat)
- Lower cardiac output (the amount of blood pumped by the heart each minute)
- Lower oxygen extraction from the blood by muscle cells
- Decreased maximal aerobic capacity (the maximal volume of oxygen the body can consume each minute)
- Blunted hormonal response
- Loss of bone mass
- Loss of muscle mass
- Fewer muscle units activated
- Reduced strength
- Slower reflexes

Within a year, Robbie will be retiring from his long career in sales management. At 66, he is looking forward to spending many healthy, active years enjoying life with his wife, who is just turning 50. Robbie realizes that the demands of his job have taken a toll on his health, body weight, and overall fitness, and he has promised himself and his wife that he'll get into better shape. He knows losing weight and getting fit will help add quality to his remaining years and perhaps extend his life as well. Robbie has lost too many friends and family members to early deaths, and he is determined to avoid the same fate. He opened a membership at a convenient fitness club and was overwhelmed by all the different class offerings and fitness equipment. He recognizes that he'll have to start slow and gradually build his strength and fitness, but he is anxious to get going. After he completes the fitness assessment at the club, he plans to try a few sessions with a personal trainer to help him get started. Robbie excitedly talks to friends and family about his fitness goals but harbors some reservations about whether he can maintain his newfound commitment over the years. For the past three decades, Robbie has allowed his health and fitness to take a backseat to his career, and he is afraid he doesn't have the discipline needed to maintain a fitness routine for the rest of his life. He realizes he'll just have to take things one day at a time and is happy that he's already started that journey.

Clarifying the Science on Physical Fitness

What Does Being Fit Actually Mean?

Since this chapter is about how to get fit and stay fit, it makes sense to include a definition so that we're all on the same page. To put it simply: Being fit is to be physically healthy and strong. Keep in mind that physical fitness is just one aspect of our overall health. According to the World Health Organization principles, "health is a state of complete physical, mental, and social well-being and not merely the absence of disease or infirmity." Because aging is associated with reduced aerobic capacity, increased fat, decreased muscle mass and strength, and compromised mobility, it's clear that aging affects our fitness and, by extension, our health. The behaviors we choose, the lifestyles we lead, how physically active we are, and what and how much we choose to eat and drink directly affect our risks of heart disease, obesity, type 2 diabetes, and even some cancers. In fact, it's estimated that 50% of all cancer deaths could be prevented if people would quit smoking, reduce alcohol consumption, maintain a healthy weight, and meet the guidelines for weekly physical activity.

Why Is Fitness So Important?

Fitness is *pleiotropic,* which is a fancy way of saying that being physically fit has many benefits for physical, mental, and social health. In fact, overall quality of life improves with weekly exercise time, as assessed by standard surveys such as the RAND Corporation-developed 36-item Short Form Health Survey, which evaluates physical functioning; emotional well-being; perceptions of energy, fatigue, and pain; and other health characteristics. Happily, it's never too late to improve our fitness; the human body is amazingly adept at increasing its fitness capacity, even in our 90s and beyond. This is why a fit 70-year-old can outperform an unfit 27-year-old. In 2016, when 100-year-old Ida Keeling broke the world record in the 100-yard dash for women over the age of 80, she was quoted as saying that her advice was to eat for nutrition, not for taste; to do what we need to do, not what we want to do; and to exercise at least once every day. Interestingly, Ida did not start running until she was 67 years old.

An often-overlooked benefit of physical activity is that the resulting increase in appetite makes it more likely that you'll eat enough to meet your daily needs of important micronutrients, macronutrients, and phytonutrients, which are the thousands of different healthy compounds found in foods like fruits, vegetables, and whole grains.

At any age, the biggest health benefits occur whenever those who are in the lowest category of fitness become physically active. This shouldn't be too surprising because the least fit have the most to gain, but it is reason enough to encourage anyone who is unfit to begin to move more each and every day.

Factors that Influence Fitness

Our interest in and capacity for improved fitness is determined by a mix of psychosocial dynamics; bone health; joint disorders; diseases and health issues of various sorts; and our current fitness, genetics, and training program design; along with personal goals and interests. The fact that you are reading this section indicates that you are interested in maintaining or improving your fitness, so that interest alone is a step in the right direction. All too often, however, those first steps don't last long because many people attempt to do too much too soon, resulting in stiffness, soreness, or sometimes an injury, which can make sitting at home seem preferable to being active. Regardless of the challenges we may face, there are easy ways to gradually and painlessly increase our daily activity and improve our fitness. There's no doubt that current health issues can limit what and how much we are able to do in terms of physical activity, but improvement is always possible.

Fitness, Health, and Disease

Rebecca is a 72-year-old woman who lives alone in a retirement community but stays active with daily walks around the neighborhood, water exercises at the pool twice a week, and the occasional stop by the community fitness center to lift weights for 15 to 30 minutes in hopes of toning her muscles. Rebecca hasn't suffered any serious health setbacks and wants to avoid such problems for as long as she can. She knows that being fit will help, but she also knows that she could—and should do—more to improve her strength and fitness. Rebecca enjoys her walks and other physical activities but isn't one for formal fitness classes; her water exercise sessions are about as much group activity as she cares for. She realizes that as she ages, her current activity level will be tough to maintain unless she improves her strength and fitness in the near future. Rebecca has seen how quickly older people can deteriorate physically and mentally, especially when they are unfit. She's willing to do more but wants to spend her fitness time efficiently. Rebecca has promised herself to learn more from her fitness center about other ways she can stay active and improve her fitness.

Being fit can help prevent early death. In fact, being unfit is a bigger risk factor for early death than being obese. In other words, it's better to have extra fat and be fit than to be thin and unfit; statistics show that fit people who are overweight live longer than unfit thin people (but remember that there are other risks with carrying extra body fat). That single benefit should be enough to motivate us to at least meet the current weekly physical activity guidelines.

Regular physical activity has more overall health benefits than the most powerful drugs. We've touched on the vast array of benefits to our physical health, but exercise also benefits mental health. People who are more physically active are less likely to suffer from cognitive decline and dementia, perhaps because regular physical activity helps maintain greater brain volume. Being fit also increases self-esteem and reduces anxiety and depression. Many people are surprised to learn that for those suffering from depression, regular exercise can be more effective than drugs at reducing symptoms. This is particularly important for those recovering and rehabbing from major surgery, when getting down in the dumps is very common. Research from the US National Institute on Aging shows that exercise boosts memory by stimulating the growth of brain cells. We know the brain communicates with and controls muscles, but muscles—especially active muscles—communicate with the brain and other tissues. During physical activity, muscles release hundreds of different compounds into the bloodstream. Those compounds can be taken up by other tissues; for instance, a compound called cathepsin B appears to stimulate the positive effects on memory associated with regular exercise, although numerous other brain-stimulating compounds will undoubtedly be found in years to come.

Confronting Myths About Physical Fitness

MYTH: Getting into shape hurts.

REALITY: Unless you're training hard for a competitive event, exercise shouldn't hurt, as in the painful kind of hurt. If you're starting a new exercise program, there is bound to be some stiffness and soreness as your muscles and joints begin to adapt, but those symptoms should be tolerable, a passing annoyance. If you experience sharp or persistent pain, see your physician.

MYTH: Improving fitness takes a lot of time.

REALITY: If you can spare 10 minutes three times each day (or 15 minutes twice each day or 30 minutes once a day), that's enough time to get into better shape, provided you exercise at a moderate intensity. Get your heart rate up, break a sweat, push your body slightly beyond what's it's used to, and your fitness will improve.

MYTH: Menopause makes it more difficult to exercise.

REALITY: Menopause makes it more important to exercise but not more difficult. Regular physical activity combats many of the changes that accompany menopause, especially loss of bone and muscle mass.

MYTH: Older adults shouldn't exercise in the heat.

REALITY: One of the benefits of being fit is that we become more tolerant of the heat. As we become more fit, we become better able to cope with heat stress, which is also cardiovascular stress because of the demands hot weather places on the heart to deliver blood to the skin to speed heat loss. Just remember that as you become more fit and better able to tolerate the heat, you also have to drink more fluids to replace sweat losses. For those who have heart disease, avoiding hot-weather activity, by exercising in the mornings or in a cooler indoor environment, is a wise precaution to reduce unnecessary stress on the heart.

MYTH: Taking 10,000 steps every day ensures adequate fitness.

REALITY: The target of 10,000 steps is just one estimate of what constitutes adequate movement during the day. Wearable monitors are of questionable accuracy in monitoring steps, distance, and heart rate but can be helpful in promoting behavior change, especially with those new to a fitness regimen. If you enjoy the feedback a wearable monitor provides, by all means use one to help you keep track of your daily activity, but keep in mind that how you look and feel can be just as important as what a monitor or scale tells you. Also, be aware that the calorie-burning values displayed on exercise equipment, such as treadmills and elliptical trainers, are simply rough estimates of energy expenditure and may be highly inaccurate.

MYTH: Monitoring heart rate during exercise is the only way to get into better shape.

REALITY: Keeping track of how much your heart rate increases during physical activity can be a good way to ensure that you're doing enough to gain a benefit, but monitoring heart rate is not the only way to gauge exercise intensity. An easier, no-cost method is to simply rate how hard the physical activity feels to you on a scale of 0 to 10. If 0 is sitting still and 10 is working as hard as you possibly can, moderate-intensity exercise is a 3 or 4; vigorous exercise is a 5 to 8; and all-out, run-for-your-life intensity is a 9 or 10.

For those who like to track their heart rate during exercise, the recommended intensity for improved fitness is from 55% to 90% of maximal heart rate (HRmax). Estimating your HRmax is easy, and this is a good formula:

$$\text{HRmax} = [208 - (0.7 \times \text{age})]$$

Using that formula, the maximal heart rate for a 62-year-old person would be as follows:

$$[208 - (0.7 \times 62)] \text{ or } 208 - 43 = 165 \text{ beats per minute}$$

Keep in mind that this formula simply *estimates* your maximal heart rate. Your actual maximal heart rate may be higher or lower, but this estimate provides a good starting point. Once you have an estimate of your HRmax, determining your target exercise heart rate is easy. If your HRmax is estimated to be 165 beats per minute, simply multiply that by 0.55 and 0.9 to determine your recommended heart rate range to exercise at 55% to 90% of HRmax. In this example, the recommended range is 91 to 149 beats per minute.

MYTH: Walking isn't exercise because it doesn't increase heart rate much.

REALITY: As we grow older, walking is a great way to improve health, lose weight, and, yes, become more fit. Walking at 3+ mph (20 minutes per mile or faster) has been shown to increase fitness, reduce blood pressure, spark weight loss, improve bone health, and reduce the risks of heart disease and depression. In addition, walking at 3+ mph will keep us out in front of the Grim Reaper, according to Australian scientists who calculated the average and maximal walking speeds associated with a reduced risk of death. The researchers reported that the Grim Reaper prefers a walking speed of 2 mph but can accelerate to 3 mph on occasion. Therefore, walking at a brisk—not leisurely—pace that raises heart rate and breathing appears to be enough to reduce the risk of early death, provided we walk regularly and meet the weekly guidelines for physical activity (150 minutes each week of moderate-intensity activity or 75 minutes of vigorous-intensity activity).

MYTH: I don't have the time to exercise.

REALITY: We're all familiar with the aggravations of a hectic life, but there is simply no excuse for not making time for physical activity, even if that activity is a short walk or a quick session with weights or calisthenics. Microworkouts that last 10 minutes or less are becoming popular for those who have difficulty finding a block of time during the day for a traditional exercise session. Hundreds of smartphone apps and online videos are available to guide us through brief (and longer) bouts of physical activity. Remember, just being active for 10 minutes three times each day at a moderate-to-high intensity level is enough to meet the minimum goals for physical activity.

MYTH: Older people should avoid high-intensity training.

REALITY: It's common for most of us to let exercise intensity slip as we get older. It's much more comfortable to exercise at a lower intensity level, especially if we're not training for a competitive event. But it turns out that exercise intensity is much more important than exercise volume (duration) when it comes to health and fitness improvement. Intense exercise, such as high-intensity interval training (HIIT), where it's difficult to say even a few words during bouts of hard effort lasting between 20 to 60 seconds, for 75 minutes each week (15 minutes, 5 days each week) results in similar health and fitness benefits to spending twice as long exercising at a lower intensity. Intense exercise isn't for everyone, but if that type of training appeals to you, build up to it gradually to make sure you won't aggravate any preexisting health or joint issues. See the next myth for more information on how to incorporate HIIT.

MYTH: High-intensity interval training is only for competitive athletes.

REALITY: In his book *The One-Minute Workout*, Martin Gibala, PhD, describes research he and others have conducted that clearly demonstrates that it doesn't take a lot of time to get in better shape. Training at high intensity is a shortcut to improved fitness and health. But HIIT is not for everyone; high-intensity activity is demanding and periodically uncomfortable. (If you have a heart condition, experience bouts of dizziness, or have joint pain, HIIT may not be the right activity for you. If you're unsure, check with your physician.) On the 0-to-10 exertion scale mentioned earlier, HIIT exercise intensity falls into the 9 to 10 range: very intense, but only for brief chunks of time. Fortunately, there are endless ways to build up the intensity of an exercise session. HIIT training can be accomplished using whatever activity you most enjoy. Here are two examples:

- Complete a 5-minute (or longer) treadmill warm-up at a comfortable speed, then increase the treadmill speed and elevation to a brisk walk up an incline that can barely be maintained for 30 seconds. After 30 seconds, decrease the speed and elevation to comfortable levels and continue walking for 2½ minutes (or more, if needed.) Repeat four to six times. The goal during the 30-second intense efforts is to raise your heart rate and tire your leg muscles. These brief efforts should be noticeably more intense than what you are used to doing. This same type of workout can be done on an elliptical trainer, a stationary cycle, a rowing machine, or in the pool.
- Using the same format of 20 to 30 seconds of high-intensity effort followed by 2 to 3 minutes of less-intense activity, engage in basic calisthenics, such as jumping jacks, burpees, push-ups, and sit-ups, as the high-intensity activities, and jog or walk in place during the low-intensity breaks.

MYTH: Exercising every day will produce the best results.

REALITY: While it's important for us to be physically active every day, it's not important to exercise hard each and every day. Doing so inevitably leads to injury, burnout, and persistent fatigue. Most elite athletes follow strict training programs that are designed to gradually improve their sports-related fitness and skills. How elite athletes go about their training offers important lessons for the rest of us. One of those lessons is to regularly vary the intensity and duration of our workouts. Not even the fittest athlete is able to train hard every day of the week, so effective training programs are designed to mix things up. For example, a week's training might include a mix of 3 days of hard training, 2 days of moderate-intensity training, 1 day of active rest, and 1 day of complete rest. Remember, exercise is the stimulus for our bodies to change. Recovery between exercise sessions, along with days of light exercise or complete rest, are needed to facilitate those changes. The box below provides a simple overview of the stimulus-facilitation-response paradigm.

How the Body Gradually Responds to Regular Physical Activity

Stimulus for Common Exercises	Facilitation	Response
Walking	Sleep/rest	Improved cardiovascular fitness
Jogging	Nutrition	Increased strength
Cycling	Hydration	Greater muscle mass
Swimming		Less body fat
Strength training		

MYTH: Stretching for 10 minutes before exercise reduces injuries.

REALITY: Sports scientists, athletic trainers, and sports medicine physicians are still trying to determine if stretching before exercise decreases the risk of injury, increases the risk, or has no effect whatsoever. While those experts continue their quest, we can conclude that maintaining good flexibility as we age is an important element in overall fitness, a topic covered in more detail in Chapter 7. Common sense and experience indicate that injuries are more likely to occur in parts of the body that have limited range of motion or weak muscles. Most of us are more likely to strain our lower backs bending to pick up something off the floor than to injure ourselves during an exercise session. Improper movement techniques, weak muscles, and limited flexibility conspire to increase injury risk. Even if proper stretching does little or nothing to prevent injuries during exercise, some stretching should be part of warming up to get your body ready for more intense activity. Stretching can also be part of your cool-down routine following a workout, when muscles are warmer and more pliable.

MYTH: Abdominal exercises are great for reducing belly fat.

REALITY: From both an aesthetic and a health perspective, excess belly fat—abdominal adipose tissue—is not good. People with large waistlines are at greater risk of metabolic syndrome—low levels of the good high-density lipoprotein cholesterol and higher levels of blood triglycerides, blood pressure, and blood glucose—a condition that predisposes them to cardiovascular disease and diabetes. Unfortunately, sit-ups and other abdominal exercises do little to reduce belly fat, simply because abdominal exercises don't burn many calories (but they can help to build underlying muscle). Fat loss in the belly and elsewhere in the body occurs when we expend enough energy (calories) to create a deficit; in other words, when we expend more calories than we ingest. Whenever that deficit occurs, the body breaks down stored fat to meet its energy needs. The best way to expend a lot of calories is through aerobic exercises, such as walking, jogging, running, cycling, and swimming.

MYTH: Yoga is a great way to lose weight.

REALITY: Yoga—in all its various forms—counts as physical activity because practicing yoga increases heart rate and metabolism and helps develop muscle strength, flexibility, balance, improved posture, and bone strength, not to mention the brain-health benefits associated with relaxation and physical activity. Although there isn't a lot of good research that illustrates the health benefits of yoga, we can assume that those benefits would be similar to those of walking and similar low-intensity activities. But because low-intensity activities don't burn a lot of calories, yoga is not a go-to activity for fat loss. If you enjoy yoga, by all means continue, but if fat loss is a goal, supplement your yoga sessions with other forms of aerobic exercise that burn more calories.

MYTH: Those new to exercise programs are at greater risk of sudden death.

REALITY: Renowned newspaper editor William Allen White famously joked, "I take my only exercise acting as a pallbearer at funerals of my friends who exercise regularly." That's a funny quote, and it's not entirely untrue. Some people do die during exercise, and the risk increases with age and with exercise intensity level. But research consistently shows that the extremely low risk of sudden death during and soon after exercise is far outweighed by the health benefits of regular physical activity. Many cases of sudden death occur because of undiagnosed—heart disease—another reminder of the importance of regular physical exams. Dying quickly might be a nice way to go out after a long and healthy life, but premature sudden death from heart disease does not fit that description!

Commonly Asked Questions About Physical Fitness

What's the difference between physical activity and exercise?

Most people think of exercise as a planned activity conducted alone or as part of a group with the goal of improving some aspect of fitness. Physical activity is often thought of as movements associated with walking, gardening, mowing the lawn, housework, and similar tasks. Our belief is that these distinctions are of little practical importance in terms of health and happiness. After all, spending an afternoon raking leaves is a whole-body workout, and mowing the lawn on a summer day is often more taxing than a neighborhood walk of the same distance. The most important lesson to keep in mind is to minimize sedentary time each day; it doesn't matter if you accomplish that with physical activity or with exercise.

Do older adults still need aerobic conditioning after age 70?

Improving and maintaining aerobic fitness is a goal at any age. Having the stamina to live the life you desire requires that you remain physically active. Getting out of breath and breaking a sweat isn't just for younger people. People of all ages can benefit from regular physical activity.

Does tai chi or qigong count as aerobic exercise?

Our firm belief is that any physical activity, aside from sleeping or sitting, counts toward maintaining good health. Sticklers for definitions might say that aerobic exercise involves only those activities that sufficiently raise heart rate and require enough muscular effort to produce measurable changes in aerobic fitness. Although tai chi, qigong, yoga, and other low-intensity activities do not result in large improvements in aerobic fitness, they can be great stepping stones to activities that do improve aerobic fitness.

Having the Confidence to Make a Fitness Plan Work for You

Physical activity promotes adaptations from head to toe because activity is a dose of stress that prompts our bodies to respond and adapt. Following established physical activity guidelines is a great way to begin to become more fit, lose excess weight, gain strength, and improve your health. Once those basic activity goals are achieved, you can set your sights on other fitness-related objectives, if that's appealing. For example, many older adults enjoy traveling, yet poor fitness can reduce the joy of visiting new places. Simply having the strength and stamina to walk through parks and cities without getting winded goes a long way toward creating enjoyable memories. And sometimes you have to lift your suitcase to cram it into the overheard bin or carry it up and down train staircases.

A great shortcut to your fitness and weight-loss goals is to take advantage of every opportunity to move your body. Getting off the couch during television commercials is one good example. Other tips people find helpful include the following:

- Exercise with friends or pets.
- Park your car farther away from work and stores to promote extra walking.

- Stand periodically at your chair during meetings.
- Set your phone alarm as a reminder of how long you've been sitting.
- During movies and travel, regularly flex your arms, stomach, back, and legs.
- Listen to your favorite music while you are exercising.
- Watch your favorite television shows or a movie while you are exercising.
- Exercise outdoors when possible.
- Find simple ways to chart your progress.
- Make a plan for exercise, along with options if your plan doesn't work.
- Don't be afraid to start small and gradually increase intensity and duration to develop new behaviors that you'll be able to sustain for the rest of your life.

Conversation with an Expert

Janet Walberg Rankin, PhD, is a professor in the Department of Human Nutrition, Foods, and Exercise at Virginia Tech, where she has been teaching and conducting research for almost 35 years. Now in her early 60s, her reasons for being physically active have changed. Janet explains:

> Earlier in my life, weight control was my primary reason for being physically active, but today, a desire to maintain health and simply feel good has become more important. That doesn't mean I ignore my weight, but it is less important to me than staying healthy and slowing the consequences of aging. I have also found that exercise boosts my mental outlook; it helps relieve mental stress or that "down" feeling we all experience every once in a while. Remembering this encourages me to get out to exercise even when I don't feel very energetic—I know I will feel better afterward.

Janet likes road cycling, swimming, and hiking for aerobic exercise and adds Body Pump and Pilates classes to maintain muscle and bone health. Janet offers three pieces of advice to others to stay physically active:

> Schedule, socialize, [and] focus on feelings. First, I put my tentative exercise schedule on my electronic calendar and plan around it. Having a regular activity schedule reduces the need to look for an elusive "free time" opening. Second, doing activities with others has always helped me be consistent. If I am meeting someone for a bike ride, I am unlikely to bail out. Physically active hobbies add social richness to my life and keep me engaged. Finally, I focus on how I will feel just after the exercise rather than on whether I'll live a few more days. This immediate reward encourages me more than just hoping I will have long-term benefits.

Janet's eating pattern supports her exercise goals. Her recent diagnosis with an endocrine disorder makes following a low-sodium diet a priority, so she adopted the lower-sodium Dietary Approaches to Stop Hypertension (DASH) eating plan, which is focused on fruits, vegetables, whole grains, fish, nuts, and dairy. Janet says, "I do splurge at times but always try to make up for it in the next meal or day. And I find it easier to eat fruits and vegetables in the summer months when the markets are rich with beautiful, fresh produce."

How the Authors Stay Fit

Chris: One of the joys of retirement and moving into part-time work is the added time to devote to being physically active. I walk my dogs 2 miles most mornings and attend a 60-minute dance aerobics class at the local YMCA three times a week. I love the social aspect of group classes, even though I lack coordination for many of the dance moves! I also play golf (poorly) at least once a week. I live on a lake, and in the summer, I like to swim between two docks, doing various strokes to get a good workout for arms, legs, and lungs. I also like active vacations; one of my major goals is to be able to travel and enjoy hiking and walking wherever I go. My husband and I have taken several cycling vacations in Europe; biking 25 to 35 miles per day is not only a great way to see the country but it also makes the wonderful food and glass of wine at the end of day even more enjoyable. I plan to gradually up my exercise intensity because my goal is to stay ahead of that Grim Reaper walking speed discussed in this chapter!

Bob: To make sure I get a minimum of 150 minutes of exercise each week, I try to complete at least three 1-hour training sessions with the local Masters swim team and on my own at the YMCA. I also like to bicycle with my wife and friends whenever we have the chance. My goal is to get at least 7 hours of a mix of moderate- and high-intensity exercise (including two to three sessions of HIIT and two sessions of strength training) each week. There are weeks when I fall short, but that doesn't bother me because those lulls give my body a chance to recover and adapt. On those occasions when I exercise too little and eat too much—and become exasperated at my lack of self-discipline—I remind myself that those times will be followed periods where I exercise too much and eat too little, so it all seems to balance out. On a daily basis, I try to keep from fooling myself about how many calories I've actually expended during my workouts, knowing that overestimating leads to overeating.

Useful Resources

Websites

Centers for Disease Control and Prevention (www.cdc.gov/physicalactivity/basics/older_adults/index.htm)

▷ *Information on the importance of staying physically active, along with links to related resources*

Go4Life from the National Institute on Aging (https://go4life.nia.nih.gov/exercises/endurance)

▷ *Online resource for those who want to find simple ways to increase daily aerobic activity, along with heart rate and breathing tips*

National Institute on Aging (www.nia.nih.gov/health/publication/exercise-physical-activity/introduction)

▷ *Practical advice for making physical activity a priority*

Physical Activity Guidelines for Americans (https://health.gov/paguidelines/guidelines)

▷ *Detailed information on the official US government suggestions for weekly physical activity goals, including a chapter on active older adults*

SilverSneakers Fitness Program (www.silversneakers.com)

▷ *A useful resource to see if you qualify for free membership at a local health club*

Books

Bits & Bytes: A Guide to Digitally Tracking Your Food, Fitness, and Health by Meagan Moyer, MPH, RDN. Chicago, IL: Eatright Press, 2017.

▷ *Tips and advice for getting started with digitally tracking food and fitness habits*

Fast After 50: How to Race Strong for the Rest of Your Life by Joe Friel. Boulder, CO: VeloPress; 2015 (www.velopress.com/books/fast-after-50)

▷ *Information and recommendations about training for peak performance for those whose competitive instincts are still strong*

The One-Minute Workout by Martin Gibala. New York, NY: Avery; 2017 (www.penguinrandomhouse.com/books/533236/the-one-minute-workout-by-martin-gibala-with-christopher-shulgan/9780399183669)

▷ *Practical tips and workout examples to get started with high-intensity interval training*

CHAPTER

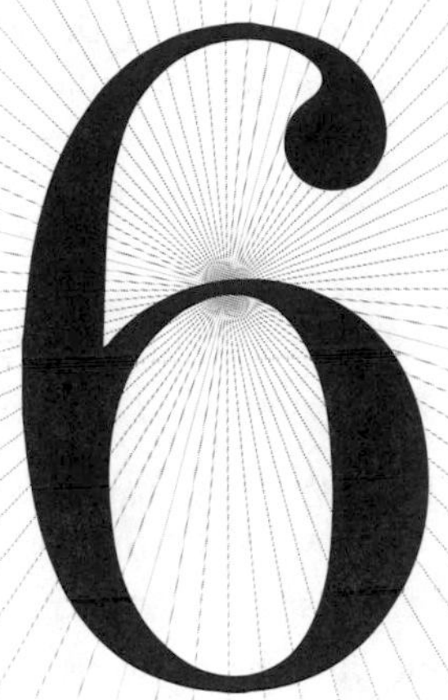

GAINING AND MAINTAINING MUSCLE AND STRENGTH

The Bottom Line

Being strong is associated with living long. Staying strong sounds reasonable and achievable, but it's complicated by the fact that all of us are challenged by a loss of muscle strength and muscle mass as we age. That's the bad news. The good news is that we can slow and sometimes reverse the loss of strength and mass by strength training at least twice each week. Here are some key points to keep in mind:

- The loss of muscle strength and mass begins around age 40, and that loss can be accelerated by a sedentary lifestyle as well as by illness and disease.
- Maintaining strength and preserving muscle mass—or at least reducing the rate at which those attributes decline—have numerous health benefits that can help us maintain functional independence well into our 90s.

- **In addition to regular strength training, consuming adequate calories (energy) and protein are important to stimulate the muscle growth that strength training promotes.**
- **Simple strength-building exercises done at home can be just as effective as training at a fitness center with expensive equipment.**

"Where did my muscles go?" Frank wondered as he looked in his bathroom mirror. Although he was never what anyone would describe as well muscled, Frank had been an athlete in high school, played intramural sports in college, and participated in local volleyball and softball leagues into his early 30s. He lifted weights on and off over the years, but those sessions became fewer and further between once he reached his 40s. Now in his late 50s, Frank is staring at a body he hardly recognizes. Muscles that seemed fairly firm when he was just a few years younger now look soft and droopy. The muscular definition that used to distinguish his shoulders from his upper arms has become indistinct, and Frank wonders how long it will be until his entire body looks like one continuous expanse of pasty flesh. Frank is certainly not alone in suddenly recognizing the age-related decline in muscle mass that is accelerated by a sedentary lifestyle. If Frank uses that realization to motivate himself to begin strength training, within months he'll be able to see improvements in his muscle mass, and perhaps he'll even lose some fat weight.

Introduction

The unfortunate fact of the matter is that as we age, we are all confronted with a decline in muscle strength, muscle mass, and muscle function. Part of the loss in muscle strength and mass is related to the aging process, but for many people, much of the decline is a culmination of decades of inactivity. As with all tissues in the body, muscles gradually adapt to their environment. If that environment is one of little physical activity, muscles slowly wither over time, reducing strength and mass, limiting basic daily activities, increasing the risk of falls and injury, and slowing recovery from illness and hospitalization.

On a positive note, if muscles are physically stressed on a regular basis, they quickly respond by increasing strength and dramatically slowing the age-related reduction in mass. Proper physical activity and nutrition combine to keep our muscles strong, so gaining knowledge and adopting practices about physical activity and nutrition can help all of us maintain health, vitality, and independence for as long as we live.

Assess Yourself: Strength

Compared with when you were 25, how do you think your strength has changed?

☐ Seems about the same
☐ Definitely weaker
☐ Definitely stronger

Compared with when you were 25, how has your muscle mass changed over time?

☐ Seems about the same
☐ Definitely less
☐ Definitely more

Compared with others my age, I feel and look stronger.

☐ Yes
☐ No

When working on my hands and knees in the yard, I can get up to my feet without a problem.

☐ Yes
☐ No
☐ I don't do yard work.

What kinds of activities do you do on a regular basis that are good for maintaining your muscle strength?

____

Which common activities, tasks, or movements do you think might now be affected by a loss of strength (such as opening jars, carrying heavy loads, or climbing stairs)?

____

I can easily lift and pour a gallon jug of milk with one hand.

☐ Yes
☐ No

I'd like to increase my muscle strength.

☐ Yes
☐ It's not an immediate concern.

I'd like to increase my muscle mass.

☐ Yes
☐ It's not an immediate concern.

Are your muscles stiff and sore when you get up in the morning?

☐ Yes
☐ No

Do your muscles get painfully sore a day or two after some activities?

☐ Yes
☐ No

Are you taking statin drugs to lower cholesterol?

☐ Yes
☐ No

Do you have any physical or medical issues that limit your strength or your ability to do resistance exercise, such as lifting weights or doing push-ups?

☐ Yes
☐ No

If yes, list the issues that limit your strength-related abilities.

____

Would you prefer to do strength exercises on your own or as part of a group?

☐ On my own
☐ As part of a group

ASSESS YOURSELF: IN REVIEW

Take the Assess Yourself quiz on the previous page before reading on.

If you responded that you are just as strong now as you were at 25, good for you! But are you sure you're not fibbing? If you had trouble coming up with examples of activities that currently help maintain your strength, that's a pretty clear indication you should add some strength training exercises to your weekly activities. And if you struggle at common movements, such as opening jars, climbing stairs, and rising from sitting to standing, that too is an indication that you can benefit from strength training. No one is promising that strength training will give you the same strength, vitality, and spring in your step that you had at 25, but strength training will definitely improve your current health and vitality.

If you struggle with limitations to your movements or are on medications that further complicate matters, there are still many options for improving muscle strength. We don't even have to leave our homes or buy equipment to get stronger. Everything we need, we already have. It's just a matter of setting aside 15 to 30 minutes at least twice each week to do strength activities that can help turn back the clock and improve our health.

By the way, if you checked "it's not an immediate concern" in response to wanting to increase strength and mass, that's reason enough to question your health and fitness goals. For all of us over 50, maintaining or increasing muscle strength and mass should be a must-do priority if we want to live long, happy, healthy, and productive lives.

James and his wife are adjusting to becoming empty nesters, as both of their sons have started their careers in different states. At 64, James is on the official countdown to retirement, an event he has mixed feelings about, although the idea of not having to adhere to a weekly work schedule is becoming more and more appealing. James's career in recreation management has long been a mixture of desk work combined with frequent short drives and walks to nearby recreation facilities to manage staff and respond to unexpected issues with equipment and grounds. He's had no major health problems, though for many years he has taken medication to control his moderately high blood pressure and cholesterol, and he is now able to ramp up his exercise routine, something that job and family responsibilities made difficult in the past. James recognizes that he could have been more physically active over the years but isn't one to fret over the past. Currently, he has been enjoying a new health club membership. He gets to the gym most days at 6 AM and completes 45 to 60 minutes of a variety of aerobic and strength training. To fill out his exercise routine, James relies on what he learned from a handful of sessions with a personal trainer and what he sees others do. He is losing weight, and he's happy with the steady progress he's making with his aerobic fitness and strength. James knows these gains will slow over time and is beginning to wonder if he'll get frustrated and bored once he reaches the point where improvements aren't as obvious. He's enjoying his newfound commitment to health and fitness, something he has promised himself to continue as he ages. He reasons that once he gets into decent shape and reaches his goal weight of 212 pounds, he'll figure out a maintenance program, one that includes enough strength training to enable him to keep up with house and yard work as well as to make it easy to accomplish the frequent hunting trips he is looking forward to.

Aging and Strength

Sarcopenia. Although the definition of the word may not immediately pop to mind (sarcopenia means "vanishing flesh"), we are all subject to its effects—the progressive loss of muscle mass, muscle strength, and muscle function as we age (see the box on page 158 for reasons why). Our capacity to live independently and fend for ourselves on a daily basis is in large part linked to how well we preserve muscle mass as we age. The good news is that even among those who have neglected their muscle health for decades, a couple of sessions each week of simple resistance exercises can increase strength and preserve muscle mass. You may already be aware that you've lost some functional strength if you're finding it more difficult to open jars, use screwdrivers, move furniture, or climb stairs. And the image in your bathroom mirror may be a daily reminder that your muscles aren't as large or as toned as they were in younger days. While some sarcopenia is inevitable as we grow older, we do have control over the rate at which it occurs because we control our physical activity and diet.

Why We Are Susceptible to Sarcopenia as We Age

- Moving less and sitting more, or engaging in exercise that's not long or intense, can lead to muscle loss. In particular, some adults do little to no strength training, the primary impetus for retaining muscle mass. To make matters worse, inactivity lowers blood flow and reduces nutrient delivery to muscles.
- With aging comes internal "wear and tear" on muscle cells. For example, decades of oxidative stress impairs muscle function and growth. Oxidative stress refers to reactions inside cells that damage proteins and other molecules. Some oxidative stress is normal, but if it isn't adequately counterbalanced, damage can gradually build and impede the normal functions of muscle cells.
- Prolonged, low-level inflammation that occurs as we age and poor health habits can interfere with normal cell function and can lead to the early death of some muscle cells.
- Age-related changes in hormone secretion leads to a loss of muscle mass (existing muscle cells shrink in size).
- Mitochondrias, the parts of the cell where carbohydrates and fats are processed to produce energy, lose some of their function, robbing muscle cells of the energy needed to maintain mass.
- Poor or reduced eating leads to insufficient energy (calories) or protein, which can limit muscle growth and repair. Added to that is the anabolic resistance that comes as we get older, as muscle cells become less able to take up and use the amino acids provided by protein foods.

In the United States, 5% of 65-year-olds are affected by sarcopenia, and that number rises to 50% in those over 80. In fact, between the ages of 20 and 90, we can lose over 50% of our muscle mass due to sarcopenia and a sedentary lifestyle. The effects of sarcopenia are slightly greater in women because their muscle mass is lower, as is their daily energy (calorie) and protein intake.

Unfortunately, loss of muscle mass and strength can occur quickly, even in younger people. For example, being confined to bed with an illness or after surgery results in a loss of 1% of muscle mass each day. The body is pretty quick at getting rid of what it perceives it no longer needs.

Our muscle mass peaks around age 25, remains more or less unchanged through roughly age 40, and then decreases about 1% each year through age 65, when the rate of decline gradually increases to 1.5% per year by age 80. Fortunately, growing older doesn't have to mean growing weaker or less healthy. Much of the age-related change in strength and mass can be prevented or at least slowed substantially by regular strength training.

Although maintaining muscle mass is an important goal as we age, so is maintaining muscle strength, especially the functional strength needed to perform common daily tasks. Opening packages and food containers, turning doorknobs, climbing stairs, and simply getting up from a chair and walking are activities that most of us don't even think about when we're younger. But as we age, even these simple movements can be severely compromised by loss of muscle strength. Research shows that 70-year-olds are about 30% weaker than they were at age 50. That's a large drop in strength over just 20 years. The decline in strength, like the loss of muscle mass, begins around age 40 but progresses more rapidly, at roughly 2% to 4% each year. Contrary to what those numbers suggest, the declines in muscle mass and strength don't occur in a linear fashion. Prolonged periods of increased sedentary time, along with periodic illnesses and hospitalizations, can accelerate the loss of muscle mass, strength, and functional capacity. At the risk of being overly repetitive, all of these changes can be slowed or prevented by the right combination of nutrition and exercise.

Felicia can feel herself losing strength; each time she looks in the mirror, she is reminded that she is losing muscle mass. Even though she's only in her late 50s, Felicia is beginning to struggle with opening some containers and feels her legs burn after climbing only a couple of flights of stairs. Felicia has ignored those signs for the past few years, telling herself that changes in product packaging and her hectic life explain the weakness in her hands and legs. She's recently realized that struggling to keep up with her husband on short bicycle rides means more than just being out of cycling shape because her leg strength wanes well before she gets out of breath. Now that's she's acknowledged that loss of strength has become an issue, Felicia is determined to do something about it; she knows things will only get worse unless she intervenes. With a full-time job and housework to accomplish, Felicia doesn't have a lot of extra time to devote to strength training, so she is looking for efficient and enjoyable ways to improve her strength and tone her muscles. Finding time to go a health club or YMCA is out of the question for Felicia. She's simply too busy. But she will begin to do some exercises at home, just after she wakes up, and again sometime during the day. Felicia recognizes that she'll need to do more over time but is happy that she's headed in that direction.

As Felicia has experienced, and as you can see in the box on the opposite page, our muscles will change as we age, and these changes can be accelerated or delayed by the right combination of nutrition and exercise. It shouldn't be surprising that a sedentary lifestyle, advanced age, and certain medications—along with illness, disease, and hospitalization—all accelerate loss of muscle strength and mass. But studies on octogenarian athletes show that physically fit, well-nourished people show much lower rates of decline in strength and mass. Putting aside science, for a moment, the real test of adequate muscle strength is how well older adults can handle basic functional movements, such as smoothly transitioning from sitting in a chair to standing up and walking, effortlessly climbing stairs, and balancing on one foot.

Clarifying the Science on Strength

Why Are Muscle Strength and Mass So Important?

We've all felt the muscular weakness that comes with a cold or flu, so we know firsthand how debilitating strength loss can be, even

How Muscle Changes as We Age

- Muscle mass is lost, especially in the fast-twitch muscle cells that support quick movements. Those cells either shrink considerably or die.
- Leg and buttock muscles lose mass, likely because we do less walking and more sitting.
- Nerve transmission to muscles slows.
- Connections between nerves and muscles deteriorate.
- Fewer muscle cells are recruited during movements, and that reduces strength.
- The process of contraction is impaired.
- Protein synthesis in muscle slows.
- Muscles become less responsive to protein in the diet (called "anabolic resistance").
- Tendons that attach muscle to bone lose some of their water content and become stiffer.

when that loss is only temporary. Having strong muscles is of great benefit when we need to rebound quickly from inevitable illnesses and accidents. It shouldn't be surprising that our strength is linked to our survival; research shows that stronger people tend to live longer. In addition, strong muscles and the vitality they provide make life more enjoyable, increasing our capacity to get the most out of each and every day. The good news is that it's never too late to improve muscle strength, and the human body is amazingly adept at increasing its strength and mass, even into our 90s. In a very real sense, resistance training can reverse some of the aging process, at least in skeletal muscle.

Hector is 76 and enjoys his life in a sunny retirement community. His beloved wife passed away 2 years ago, and after getting over that devastating loss, Hector has begun to rediscover his strong love of living. An entire year of being emotionally down in the dumps also took a physical toll because Hector spent a lot of time just sitting in his house, occasionally doing odd chores and periodically hosting one of his four children and their families when they came to visit. Hector never had to worry about staying fit because he worked his entire life in the construction industry, first framing houses and then steadily moving up the ranks to become a site supervisor and then project manager. Even when his job required less manual labor, Hector still stayed active almost every day at work, scrambling up and over job sites to inspect the work and talk to the crew. After he retired, Hector and his wife enjoyed taking long walks through the neighborhood, going to the community gym a couple of times each week to lift weights and use the resistance machines, and swimming in their pool and at the local beaches. Hector knows his physical capacity has declined, and he is particularly concerned about the loss of strength and muscle tone that have occurred since his wife's death. He was always one of the strongest guys on any job site, and he was proud of that. Now it's time to regain some of that strength, but Hector hardly knows how to begin. His strength always came naturally, not as a result of working out. Hector realizes he now has to develop new lifestyle habits that include regular strength training sessions. He knows a few guys in his neighborhood who use a personal trainer and plans to contact them to learn more. Hector understands that he needs some help to get his new routine started, and that then he can rely on his natural motivation to keep it going.

There are many benefits associated with maintaining muscle strength and mass—including helping us live healthy, happy, independent lives for as long as possible. This list should be an incentive for all of us to make certain that regular strength training (at least twice each week) is part of our regimen (see the box on the oppposite page). Hector was blessed by his genetics with natural strength, but even he will have to work to maintain that strength and his muscle mass as he ages. That's good for Hector because there is a strong connection between being strong and living long.

Benefits You Can Expect from Strength Training and Healthy Eating

- Stabilized arthritic joints
- Improved balance
- Reduced risk of falls
- Increased resting metabolism
- Improved appearance
- Increased social interactions
- Lowered risk of all-cause mortality
- Lowered risk of diabetes
- Lowered risk of osteoporosis
- Lowered risk of low back pain
- Lowered risk of obesity
- Accelerated recovery from illness and surgery
- Improved sleep
- Reduced incidence of depression
- Enhanced self-esteem
- Improved self-confidence
- Enhanced overall well-being

What Does Being Strong Actually Mean?

It's obvious that in virtually all sports, improving muscle strength is an important part of improving performance. Athletes strive to improve—or at least maintain—strength over the course of a season or a career. But those strength improvements have to be functionally relevant. For example, strength is an important characteristic for baseball pitchers, but it doesn't make much sense for pitchers to develop the physique or strength of bodybuilders. Improved strength has to contribute to improved pitching. The same is true as we age; we have to maintain the functional strength that enables us to enjoy the lives we desire.

When we were younger, it was easy to take our muscles for granted. Our muscles were just there, and they usually did what we asked of them. Stiff, sore, weak, uncooperative muscles were the exception, not the rule. Whenever we asked our muscles to perform a task, they did so obediently. As we age, that obedience begins to waver in small, almost imperceptible ways at first, before slowly regressing over the years to what might feel at times like a full-scale revolt.

Skeletal muscles are basically motors that move bones around joints. Individual muscles—for example, the biceps muscle that flexes the arm—comtain hundreds of thousands of individual muscle cells, each with the capacity to contract when called upon by the nervous system to do so. Those individual muscle cells are arranged into units ranging from only ten to over a thousand cells, each unit controlled by a nerve connected to the spinal cord and brain. When that nerve fires, all the muscle cells connected to it contract simultaneously. Need to pick a pen up from the desk? That's easily accomplished by activating just a few nerve–muscle units (scientists refer to these as motor units.). Need to pick up a 40-pound bag of compost while you're working in the yard? That too can be accomplished by activating many more nerve–muscle units to create the force needed to lift the bag.

You may have already figured out that muscle strength depends in part on how many nerve–muscle units can be activated, as well as by the force that can be produced by each tiny muscle cell. We can gain strength by activating more nerve–muscle units and by increasing the size—and therefore the force—of individual muscle cells. Both of those changes occur with strength training.

Factors that Influence Strength

Skeletal muscle is an extremely plastic tissue, meaning that muscle cells—and the nerves that connect to them—adapt quickly to the requirements of life. If those requirements are meager, our muscles slowly shrink in size—they atrophy and lose some of their functional capacity. Most of us have experienced how just a few days of being confined to bed affects muscle strength, and longer stints in bed have a noticeable impact on muscle mass. In fact, just 2 weeks of taking fewer than 1,000 steps each day results in reduced muscle protein synthesis, a loss of lean body mass (water, muscle, and bone), and impaired muscle function.

Fortunately for all of us, even muscles atrophied by many years of a sedentary lifestyle can regain strength and mass if they are stimulated by regular exercise to do so. That's why staying physically active, including at least 2 days each week of some sort of strength training, is part of the current US Physical Activity Guidelines, recommendations that become increasingly important as we age.

Optimal gains in strength and mass are associated with exercising muscles to failure at least two times each week. "To failure" might have caught your attention because that sounds unpleasant. In this case, failure refers to exercising until your muscles stop cooperating. For some people, that could mean lifting until they are unable to lift the weight one more time; in other words, complete but temporary muscle fatigue. Failure can also mean lifting a weight until you can feel your muscles begin to quiver and lose coordination from the effort. Fortunately, there are a wide variety of ways to strengthen muscles, and it's not always necessary to exercise them to failure. After all, truly fatigued muscles can be downright painful, so on days that you aren't mentally prepared for a little discomfort, simply completing a strength-training routine will be good enough.

Confronting Myths About Muscle Strength

MYTH: It's difficult for older people to gain strength and mass.

REALITY: Nonsense. One of the marvelous things about muscle is that it is quick to adapt to strength training. In fact, your strength will increase soon after you begin training, not because your muscle cells have gotten larger but because your nervous system is the first to adjust to the new demands.

MYTH: The only way to tone muscles is to lift heavy weights.

REALITY: Toning muscles occurs as a combination of an increase in the size of the muscle and a reduction in the thickness of the fat that lies between muscle and skin. Lifting heavy weights is a good way to achieve both of those changes, but it's not the only way. Lifting lighter weights for more repetitions (eg, doing three sets of 20 repetitions of bicep curls) will be just as effective, provided your muscles get as tired as they would if they were lifting heavier weights.

MYTH: Aerobic training reduces muscle strength.

REALITY: This is the kind of statement that looks like it would be simple to answer but isn't. We've all seen photos of elite distance runners and Tour de France cyclists whose upper bodies look like they haven't yet gone through puberty. And even their legs, as incredible as they are at powering the athletes up and down roads at inconceivable speeds, are usually well toned but thin. So one might reasonably conclude that aerobic training, especially large amounts of aerobic training, will reduce muscle strength, at least in those muscles that aren't used. And that is partially true. The loss of muscle mass in the upper body of runners and cyclists is associated with a loss of strength, but the legs, the limbs that are aerobically fit, often become stronger with training, even though they remain thin. In fact, aerobic training may actually augment the benefits of strength training by altering certain cellular responses. For those of us who do modest amounts of both aerobic and resistance exercise, the benefits for muscle strength and overall health are complementary.

MYTH: Effective strength training requires a high-protein diet.

REALITY: A high-protein diet is not required, but it can be helpful. That's particularly true for older adults because of the anabolic resistance that occurs with age. Anabolic refers to metabolic processes that build new tissue (some athletes cheat by taking anabolic steroids to speed up the muscle-building process). As we age, our muscles become less sensitive—more resistant—to the amino acids that come from the digestion and absorption of proteins in our diet. Whenever muscles are exposed to an increased amount of amino acids, their usual response is to incorporate those amino acids into proteins to aid muscle contraction and develop additional structures within muscle cells. With age, that usual response is blunted. It takes more amino acids to provoke the same amount of muscle protein synthesis.

MYTH: The current dietary guidelines for protein intake are more than sufficient for older adults.

REALITY: Get ready for a few numbers to help us explain why this is a myth. The US Institute of Medicine macronutrient guidelines have for many years identified the adequate daily protein intake as 0.36 grams of dietary protein for every pound of body weight (or 0.8

grams per kilogram) each day. For a 165-pound person, that would amount to 60 grams of protein each day. New research shows that most of us can benefit from more protein, especially as we grow older and continue our physical activity. The latest recommendations are to consume 0.55 to 0.68 grams per pound (or 1.2 to 1.5 grams per kilogram) of body weight each day. That would increase the recommended daily protein intake for a 165-pound person from 60 grams per day to between 90 and 115 grams per day, a sizable jump.

MYTH: Protein is best consumed at dinner so that the muscle cells can incorporate the amino acids during sleep.

REALITY: We Americans do indeed consume most of our daily protein intake at the evening meal. We typically consume the least amount of protein at breakfast and a modest amount at lunch, saving the largest amount for dinner. Emerging research shows that evenly spreading out our protein intake throughout the day is the best way to stimulate muscle protein synthesis and enhance the benefits of exercise. By evenly distributing protein intake throughout the day, muscles have a better chance to put all the amino acids to good use. The basic idea is to consume 0.18 to 0.23 grams of protein per pound (0.4 to 0.5 grams per kilogram) of body weight at breakfast, lunch, and dinner. For our 165-pound example person, that would mean eating 30 to 38 grams of protein at each meal, for a total of roughly 90 to 115 grams each day. The table on page 168 suggests protein ranges and amounts per meal for various weights.

RECOMMENDATIONS FOR DAILY PROTEIN INTAKE TO SUPPORT MUSCLE STRENGTH AND MASS*

Body Weight (pounds)	Protein/Meal (grams)	Total Daily Protein (grams)
100	18-23	55-68
110	20-25	61-75
120	22 -28	66-82
130	23-30	72-88
140	25-32	77-95
150	27-35	83-102
160	29-37	88-109
170	31-39	94-116
180	32-41	99-122
190	34-44	105-129
200	36-46	110-136
210	38-48	116-143
220	40-51	121-150
230	41-53	127-156
240	43-55	132-163

*It is not necessary to be precise in your protein intake. Just try to get close to the range of your body weight.

It's not necessary to be precise in your protein intake, just try to get close to the range for your body weight. See the box on page 169 for protein amounts in common foods.

PROTEIN AMOUNTS IN COMMON FOOD AND BEVERAGES

Animal Protein Foods	Protein (grams)
Chicken breast, grilled (3 ounces)	26
Beef, sirloin, broiled (3 ounces)	26
Pork loin, roasted (3 ounces)	23
Salmon, sockeye, baked (3 ounces)	23
Ground beef, 90% lean, broiled (3 ounces)	22
Tuna, canned in water (3 ounces)	20
Whey protein powder (1 ounce)	17
Cottage cheese (1/2 cup)	14
Greek yogurt, nonfat (5 ounces)	13
Milk, low fat (8 ounces)	8
Cheese, cheddar (1 ounce)	6
Egg, large (1)	6
Yogurt, regular, nonfat (5 ounces)	4
Plant Protein Foods	**Protein (grams)**
Tempeh (1/2 cup)	17
Soy nuts, dry roasted (1/4 cup)	10
Soybeans (edamame), cooked (1/2 cup)	9
Tofu, regular (1/2 cup)	9
Lentils, cooked (1/2 cup)	9
Peanut butter, creamy (2 tablespoons)	9
Kidney beans, canned, drained (1/2 cup)	8
Soy milk, 8 ounces	7
Hummus (1/3 cup)	6
Almonds (1 ounce)	6
Sunflower seeds (1 ounce)	5
Quinoa, cooked (1/2 cup)	4
Walnuts (1 ounce)	4
Bulgur, cooked (1/2 cup)	3
Pecans (1 ounce)	3
Almond milk (8 ounces)	2

To give you an idea of what a balanced protein intake might look like, the box below shows sample daily meals, each of which contains 30 grams of protein, to demonstrate how protein can be spread evenly throughout the day. Grams of protein are shown in parentheses. The table on page 169 compares the protein from several familiar protein food sources. See Chapter 2 for more about complete and incomplete protein.

SAMPLE MEALS CONTAINING 30 GRAMS OF PROTEIN

Sample Breakfast Menus		
6 ounces Greek yogurt (18) 1 ounce granola (4) Small banana (1) Nonfat milk latte (6)	2 scrambled eggs with 1 ounce cheese and spinach (21) 8 ounces soy milk (7) ½ slice whole grain toast (2)	Smoothie made with 1 ounce whey protein powder (20) 6 ounces vanilla Greek yogurt (18) ½ cup frozen berries (1)
Sample Lunch Menus		
1 cup cottage cheese (28) 1 Tablespoon chopped nuts (1) 3 slices fresh or canned peaches (1)	3 ounces tuna mixed with mayonnaise (21) 2 slices whole grain bread (7) Lettuce, tomato, banana peppers, or other veggies (2)	3 ounces cheddar cheese (21) 6 whole grain crackers (2) 8 ounces nonfat milk (8)
Sample Dinner Menus		
Large green salad with veggies and oil-and-vinegar dressing (2) 4 ounces grilled chicken or salmon (28) 1 Tablespoon sunflower seeds (1) 1 Tablespoon chopped nuts (1)	Stir fry with ½ cup tofu (10) Carrots, broccoli, and edamame (16) 1 cup brown rice (5)	1 cup pasta (6) 3 ounces turkey or beef meatballs (21) Green salad with balsamic vinegar dressing (1)

MYTH: It's impossible for older people to take in enough dietary protein without consuming special protein or amino-acid supplements.

REALITY: Consuming protein or amino-acid supplements is not necessary to meet our daily protein needs, but it can sometimes be helpful, especially when the appetite is dulled. Also consider high-protein drinks that contain 20 grams of protein or more per serving. Look for whey protein as a major ingredient because research shows that whey protein is very effective at stimulating muscle protein synthesis. Dairy foods, such as milk and yogurt, contain whey protein. For vegetarians, soy is a complete protein that also stimulates muscle protein synthesis.

MYTH: The best way to improve strength is to repeat the same exercises every week with heavier weights.

REALITY: If you have a high tolerance for boredom, this approach can be effective, but for those of us who like variety in our workouts, it's thankfully not necessary to do anything other than regularly stress our muscles at least a couple of times each week, ideally to the point where they are temporarily tired. If your muscles remain tired day after day, that's a sign you should ease off the training until they feel normal again.

MYTH: Improving strength and mass takes a lot of time.

REALITY: The great thing about strength training is that improvements come very quickly, first as a result of our nervous system recruiting more muscle cells and then as a result of increases in muscle proteins that aid contraction. The first response occurs within days, while the increase in protein synthesis occurs over weeks and months. Finding everyday ways to get stronger can make it easy to improve strength and mass. For example, taking the stairs rather than an escalator or elevator, carrying luggage on trips, rearranging furniture, planting new shrubs or flowers, walking hills in the neighborhood, and lugging groceries are examples of activities that stress our muscles and promote increased strength.

Commonly Asked Questions About Strength

Is muscle soreness required to gain strength?

A little soreness can actually be a good thing in the day or two after training. Not only is mild muscle soreness a reminder that we exercised hard enough to stimulate our muscles, but the soreness also triggers improvements in muscle that lead to greater strength and mass. Keep in mind that soreness is not required for strength gain, but it can help accelerate the growth of bigger, stronger muscles.

Is it true that using something like aspirin or ibuprofen reduces strength gains?

NSAID is the abbreviation for nonsteroidal anti-inflammatory drugs, such as aspirin, ibuprofen, and naproxen. Because of the way NSAIDs work to reduce inflammation, there was concern that they might also blunt adaptations to training. Subsequent research has shown that this is not the case.

Should I eat a special combination of foods to help add muscle strength and mass?

There is no special combination of foods that is best for adding strength and mass. Staying well hydrated, consuming adequate calories (energy), and eating enough protein with each meal are the three pillars of nutrition that support muscle protein synthesis. Consuming a protein rich meal soon after exercise is the best way to stimulate muscle cells to build new proteins. Some evidence also suggests that eating an adequate amount of omega-3 fatty acids, the polyunsaturated fatty acids in fish oil, may also support gains in muscle strength.

Will strength training cause me to gain weight and look bulky?

The propensity to gain muscle as a result of strength training is in large part determined by our genetics. Some people can gain a lot of strength with very little increase in muscle mass, while others add muscle quickly. The general rule is that if you want to gain strength and minimize the increase in mass, lift lighter weights for more repetitions (eg, instead of doing three sets of eight repetitions of a chest press with 80 pounds, do three sets of 20 reps with 30 pounds). Keep in mind that an added benefit of increasing muscle mass is that doing so boosts metabolism. First, there is a metabolic boost each time you exercise. Second, as your body adds muscle mass and reduces fat, resting metabolic rate increases because muscle cells are more metabolically active than fat cells. As a result, you can burn hundreds of additional calories each day, making it easier to keep excess weight off.

Having the Confidence to Make a Strength Training Plan Work for You

Now in her mid-50s, Ann is delighted when people tell her she looks at least 10 years younger. Looking and feeling good are important for Ann, although those goals fall much lower on her totem pole of priorities than making sure her husband's and son's needs are met. Ann is the ultimate caretaker, and putting the needs of others before herself is just part of her nature. She won't take time to exercise unless the house is clean and her loved ones don't need her immediate attention. Ann knows that as she ages, maintaining her strength and muscle mass are critical, not only for her health but also for her appearance. She's already concerned that her upper arms look a bit flabby, even though she weighs only 10 pounds more than she did in high school. Loss of muscle mass will do that, and Ann realizes she has to find a way to increase her strength training. Knowing she doesn't have the time or the inclination to spend a lot of time in the gym, Ann's goal is to find a strength program that will give the greatest benefits in the least amount of time. Ann's goals for strength training are primarily cosmetic—to reduce flabby arms and lose fat weight—but she also realizes that maintaining her strength and muscle mass will be important as she ages. Ann likes the convenience of exercising at home with light weights and tries to strength train at least twice each week, devoting just 20 to 30 minutes to each session. She is comfortable following her own routine, although periodically she and her husband work out together to exercise videos on strength training. Ann can see the skin on her arms becoming tighter as her arm muscles gradually show more tone and size, and that alone is motivation to continue.

Ann is definitely not alone in her desire to make her exercise time as efficient as possible. After all, why work out for an hour when we can accomplish the same results in 20 minutes? In fact, it's becoming more and more apparent that shorter, more intense workouts are just as effective as longer sessions. More about that approach in a bit.

Let's start with the understanding that there is no pill, potion, supplement, or exercise gizmo that provides a shortcut to improved muscle strength or mass (anabolic steroids are the exception), and there is no particular type of resistance training scheme that is best. Muscles adapt to being stressed, and there are infinite ways to accomplish just that. The best exercise equipment and the best workouts are whatever you enjoy using and will continue to use. If you think special equipment is needed to gain strength, arm wrestle a farmer sometime! Muscle strength and mass are developed whenever our muscles are overloaded on a regular basis and naturally adapt to meet those increased demands. It's really no more complicated than that.

Those who have access to a community or private fitness center, YMCA, recreation center, or nearby school or university will likely find there lots of on-site equipment and expertise to help design and implement effective strength-training programs. For those who prefer to exercise at home, personal trainers and internet resources can get you going.

Adults who are new to strength training or returning to strength training after a long hiatus should keep some basic advice in mind:

- *Always use proper technique.* If you're not sure what that is, get some advice from a trained sports health professional, such as a certified athletic trainer, a physical therapist, or a qualified personal trainer.
- *Embrace mild muscle soreness, but avoid muscle and joint pain.* For many, especially those taking a statin medications for cholesterol, mild muscle soreness is not unusual. Soreness certainly isn't unusual when we first start a new exercise program, but muscle and joint pain that makes you wince is a signal that something is not right, and it should be an impetus to seek medical attention.

- *Start light and easy; build gradually.* Many people make the mistake of trying to do too much too soon and become so sore that they soon give up on strength training. Take it easy for the first few weeks and gradually increase the number of sets, repetitions, and resistance over time.
- *Breathe correctly.* Exhale on the hard parts and inhale on the easy parts. Never hold your breath. For instance, when doing a chest press, exhale as you push the bar or dumbbell away from you, and inhale as you slowly lower it back toward you.
- *Minimize rapid eccentric movements.* Eccentric refers to movements where your muscles are lengthening at the same time they are contracting. Lowering a weight after a biceps curl is a good example of an eccentric contraction. Doing that movement too quickly or with too much resistance will damage muscle cells, resulting in a few days of pain and swelling.
- *Stand, sit, and lie down.* Challenge your muscles to operate in a variety of different positions. Numerous strength training exercises are designed to use different body positions. One often overlooked exercise that's great for all ages is to simply lie flat on your back on the floor and then move to a standing position. Do this repeatedly and experiment with different ways of getting up and returning to the floor. Your body weight is more than enough resistance to help build strength and mass, along with newfound movement skills.
- *Use one limb and both limbs.* In fancier terms, do exercises that use both unilateral (one limb) and bilateral (both limbs) movements. You can do chest presses with dumbbells using one arm at a time or use a barbell with both arms active at the same time.
- *Remember that any resistance will do.* Free weights, stretch cords, body weight, and exercise machines all offer resistance that can be used to effectively stress our muscles and produce gains in strength and mass.

Making the most efficient use of our time is important, even if we might have a lot of free time. We previously mentioned that aerobic training can also help build muscle strength. And so can high-intensity interval training (sometimes abbreviated as HIIT). This type of training (also covered in Chapter 5) takes a little getting used to but can be a very time-efficient way to squeeze in a workout if you like the challenge of exercising intensely. A HIIT workout can last as little as 15 to 30 minutes yet deliver the same benefits as sessions that are three times as long. The key element in HIIT training is repeated brief bouts of high-intensity exercise. As an example, imagine doing an easy 10-minute warm-up on a stationary cycle, followed by 20 seconds of cycling as hard as you possibly can. After those 20 seconds, you reduce your intensity back to the warm-up level and continue cycling for 2 or 3 minutes before repeating the 20-second all-out effort. Repeat that three to six times and your workout is over in less than 30 minutes. Though HIIT training is obviously not for everyone, keep it in mind as a workout option that can increase leg strength and stamina.

For those just beginning a strength-training program or those limited in what they can do, many alternative approaches are effective at increasing strength and preserving muscle mass. Many of these exercises simply use your own body weight as the resistance, although light dumbbells, stretch cords, or even cans of soup or other household items can be used to provide resistance. Take a look at the Useful Resources section on page 180 for some helpful websites for getting started with a strength-training routine.

Conversation with the Experts

Jeff Zachwieja, PhD, is senior director for Global Nutrition Sciences at PepsiCo. Now in his early 50s, Jeff is tall, lean, and athletic. The combination of the right genetic makeup, a reasonably good diet throughout his life, and a lifelong devotion to physical activity has kept his weight in check and sustained his capacity to run or swim for at least an hour most days and still have energy left over for yard work or time in his garage restoring old cars. Jeff's in-depth understanding of how nutrition and exercise combine to support a healthy, active lifestyle gives him an advantage most of us don't have: Jeff knows the underlying science and has the training and experience needed to distinguish fact from fiction.

Jeff explains:

> Making judgments about the practical implications of new research is risky because it's easy to jump the gun, only to have subsequent studies change things. This is why it seems like coffee is good for us one day and bad for us the next. It takes many studies over many years to create the confidence needed to make practical recommendations.

Working in nutrition and exercise research also gives Jeff valuable insights about how daily nutrition influences the body's responses to physical activity, especially the function of muscles. Jeff says that as he gets older, he has found that strength training and flexibility exercises are essential to maintaining his strength and muscle mass (Chapter 7 covers flexibility, balance, and agility).

Jeff considers his diet to be equally important, adding:

> Regardless of the type of exercise I do, I try to consume foods or convenience items that provide high-quality protein. I feel better when I do that, and it seems to make it easier to get through consecutive days of workouts. Even on rest days, I make sure to eat a variety of protein sources to help my muscles recover, repair, and grow.

Donald K. Layman, PhD, Professor Emeritus in the Department of Food Science and Nutrition at the University of Illinois-Urbana-Champaign has been conducting research on the role of protein in health for more than 25 years. Don says:

> My research helped me to understand the importance of balancing protein and carbohydrates at each meal. Protein research has shown that adults need more protein at each meal because we become less efficient at using protein to stimulate the necessary daily repair of our muscles as we age. We need to optimize this repair process to keep our muscles fit and strong.

Now in his mid-60s, Don practices what he teaches:

> I exercise at least 90 minutes every day. I like to play tennis three or four times each week, and the other days I do a combination of biking, running, yoga, and weightlifting. I'm a big fan of high-intensity interval training (HIIT). As I get older, the maximum intensity has gone down, but I still try to combine intensity, strength, and flexibility at every workout.

Don's motivation to stay active goes beyond the physiological reasons for exercise. He says, "I simply enjoy being active. My hobbies are tennis, snow skiing, and scuba diving, so it's important for me to stay in shape to have fun and avoid injuries. I would encourage everyone to find a combination of activities they can enjoy and can do routinely." Don's biggest concerns about aging are losing flexibility and mobility, so he invests in healthy eating and regular exercise to "maximize my potential for healthy aging."

He describes his typical dietary intake as "protein-centric" and moderates the amount of grains and starchy vegetables that he eats. He describes his typical diet as follows:

> My breakfast is based on dairy proteins, and I use whey protein, kefir, and Greek yogurt plus berries to make a high-protein shake. Adults need a minimum of 20 to 30 grams of protein at each meal for healthy muscles. Most adults get less than 12 grams at breakfast. For lunch, I emphasize fresh vegetables and protein-rich foods, including eggs, meat, and cheese. For dinner, I have meat or fish with lots of vegetables and some type of carbohydrate. My body tolerates more carbohydrates at later meals, and I avoid snacking between meals.

Don recommends if you're over 50, you should "find a daily exercise that you enjoy and causes you to stress your muscles, and start your day with a high-protein breakfast."

How the Authors Build and Maintain Muscle

Knowing the research on building and maintaining exercise is helpful, but it still takes a plan for Chris and Bob to work their muscles. Chris started strength training in her early 50s when she joined the local YMCA, which had a strength program outlined on computers at every machine to track progress. Bob knows the importance of strength training and has been doing some type of strength training for most of his adult life.

Chris: I like structure and routine, so I use the weight machines for my strength workout. I do a 20-minute circuit of 12 to 15 reps repeated three times for major muscle groups (legs, back, and arms) and add dumbbells for biceps and triceps. I don't use every machine, just leg extensions, hamstring curls, chest press and rows, pulldowns, and shoulder press. I like the machines because I can really gauge my progress when I start adding more weight to a machine. I try to weight train twice a week, but although I know it is important and I see results quickly, it is not my favorite thing to do! I aim for 20 to 25 grams of protein at meals, but, for me, lunch is the hardest meal to get protein. My favorite protein-containing foods are Greek yogurt, cottage cheese, almonds, walnuts, pistachios, pecans, peanuts, chicken or turkey breast, and tuna. On cereal, I use milk that is ultrafiltered, which means that its protein and calcium content is concentrated so that a serving has 50% more protein and 30% more calcium than regular milk.

Bob: I like variety in my strength workouts. Lifting weights session after session is just too boring. Online workout videos have been a great way to get the variety I crave, and they are still challenging enough to help maintain my muscle mass and strength. Now that I'm in my late 60s, I can see how quickly my muscle mass begins to disappear after a couple of weeks of not working out. I'm hoping that having continued variety in my workouts will help me maintain a lifelong commitment to strength training. For protein intake, I try to evenly spread it out so that I eat 30 to 40 grams of protein with each meal. That has helped me gradually increase my muscle mass and keeps me from overeating—an added bonus.

Useful Resources

American College of Sports Medicine (http://journals.lww.com/acsm-msse/Fulltext/2009/07000/Exercise_and_Physical_Activity_for_Older_Adults.20.aspx)

▷ *Expert position statement that includes the scientific background supporting fitness recommendations for older adults*

Centers for Disease Control and Prevention (www.cdc.gov/nccdphp/dnpa/physical/growing_stronger/growing_stronger.pdf)

▷ *Booklet with useful suggestions about gaining and maintaining muscle strength as we age*

Fitness Blender (www.fitnessblender.com)

▷ *Example of an online and app-based fitness program that lets visitors pick and choose among hundreds of guided workouts varying in duration and difficulty*

iMuscle2 (http://applications.3d4medical.com/imuscle2)

▷ *An app that provides information about the location, names, and functions of muscles and suggestions for strengthening and stretching individual muscles*

Go4Life from the National Institute on Aging (https://go4life.nia.nih.gov/exercises/strength)

▷ *Online resource with photo examples of simple strength-building exercises that can be done at home; especially helpful for those who are just beginning a strength-building program*

World Health Organization (www.who.int/dietphysicalactivity/factsheet_olderadults/en)

▷ *Helpful information about physical activity guidelines and the many health benefits of staying active for older adults*

CHAPTER

KEEPING YOUR BALANCE, FLEXIBILITY, AND AGILITY

The Bottom Line

Scientific evidence overwhelmingly shows that getting our bodies moving on a regular basis results in a long list of benefits that can improve longevity and our overall quality of life. We devote this chapter to balance, flexibility, and agility because they are distinct characteristics that are separate from, yet complementary to, cardiovascular fitness and muscular strength. Being more aerobically fit and feeling stronger are certainly important, but to maximize overall health benefits, we also have to ensure that our balance, flexibility, and agility are maintained.

As you are likely aware, aging and inactivity can negatively affect your balance, flexibility, and agility. As a result, the older you become, the more prone you are to falls or to pain caused by strained muscles and joints. All of these injuries can immediately hamper your ability to

live independently and enjoy the quality of life you desire. Here are a few key points to keep in mind:

- **Balance, flexibility, and agility can all be improved with regular practice and should be part of a well-designed exercise program.**
- **All too often, balance, flexibility, and agility training are neglected in favor of cardiovascular and strength training.**
- **Anything you can do to prevent injuries and falls as you age will protect your overall quality of life and your ability to stay active and injury free.**
- **If you're just beginning a commitment to improved fitness, consider starting with a few weeks of balance, flexibility, and agility training as a preface to cardiovascular and strength training.**

Juanita is nearing 75 and leads an active life that she'd like to continue for as long as possible. She and her husband, Ronnie, like to tend to their lawn and landscaping, taking pride in its appearance and their ability to keep it looking nice. When the weather permits, they spend at least an hour each day keeping up with the weeds, replacing dead plants, rearranging flower beds, and trimming where needed. Some days, they're in the yard for 3 or 4 hours and are understandably tired at the end of those days. Neither Juanita nor Ronnie participates in any regular exercise programs because they've been able to maintain their body weights and overall good health just by keeping active with yard work and neighborhood walks. Now that their children are all living on their own, there is plenty of extra time for Juanita and Ronnie to stay active outside, and their home in Arizona makes that possible all year. As they've grown older, both have noticed that it's become tougher to get up and down from the ground, and they're less agile than they used to be, often catching their feet on rocks or plants in the yard and on hikes in the surrounding hills. Those occasional mishaps concern them both because they so enjoy being outside together.

Introduction

It's easy to think of being physically fit as having muscles strong enough to accomplish daily tasks, along with the cardiovascular (aerobic) capacity to power you through the day. But other aspects of fitness are equally important, and those include maintaining the balance, flexibility, and agility that enable independent living and help prevent nagging—and sometimes life-shortening—injuries. The story of Juanita and Ronnie is one that anyone who does yard work can appreciate. Tending to flower beds requires a lot of kneeling, reaching, squatting, rising, and deftly moving from one spot to another to avoid trampling flowers and shrubs in the process. That work requires balance, flexibility, and agility, attributes that decline with age—especially among those who have done little physical activity in their adult years.

All the running, jumping, dodging, skipping, hopping, and balancing you enjoyed as a child are likely distant memories, although your nervous system still remembers the basics and can help you regain some of those atrophied skills. All you have to do is incorporate movements into your daily life to help you improve the balance, flexibility, and agility that are essential to healthy aging and independent living.

ASSESS YOURSELF: IN REVIEW

Before continuing, take the Assess Yourself quiz on the next page.

It's not unusual for balance, flexibility, and agility to decline with age. After all, most of us don't participate in activities and sports that help maintain those characteristics at more youthful levels. But when those movement skills deteriorate too much, active and independent living is threatened because of the increased risk of falls, injuries, and restricted movements, and the resulting inability to fend for ourselves on a daily basis.

Balance, flexibility, and agility wane with age mostly because we neglect them. One of the many negatives associated with a sedentary lifestyle is that overall motor function—our ability to move in unrestricted ways—atrophies along with muscle mass (discussed in

Assess Yourself: Balance, Flexibility, and Agility

What current muscle, joint, or movement problems restrict your lifestyle?

____

How long can you stand on one foot with your eyes *open* and arms at your sides before losing your balance? (Loss of balance is when your raised foot touches the floor or your other leg, you begin to hop, or you have to steady yourself with your arms.)

- ☐ More than 20 seconds
- ☐ 15 to 20 seconds
- ☐ Less than 15 seconds

How long can you stand on one foot with your eyes *closed* and arms at your sides before losing your balance? (Loss of balance is when your raised foot touches the floor or your other leg, you begin to hop, or you have to steady yourself with your arms.)

- ☐ More than 10 seconds
- ☐ 5 to 10 seconds
- ☐ Less than 5 seconds

How about balancing on your other foot? Is there a large difference in your ability to balance between feet?

- ☐ Yes
- ☐ No

When was the last time you lost your balance and fell?

____

How often have you fallen during the past 6 months?

- ☐ Only once
- ☐ Twice
- ☐ More than twice but less than five times
- ☐ Five times or more

Is one leg or ankle noticeably weaker than the other or restricted in some way?

- ☐ Yes
- ☐ No

How would you characterize your ability to walk *forward* in your house?

- ☐ Unrestricted; no problems.
- ☐ Usually there are no problems, but I am walking more slowly than when I was younger.
- ☐ I have to use a cane or walker when walking more than just around the house.

How would you characterize your ability to walk *backward* in your house?

- ☐ Unrestricted; No problems, even though I don't do it much.
- ☐ I can do it, but I move slowly and am concerned I might fall.
- ☐ I haven't walked backward for years and am not about to try now.

How would you characterize your ability to walk *sideways* in your house (either shuffling sideways or moving one foot sideways behind the other)?

- ☐ Unrestricted; no problems, even though I don't do it much.
- ☐ I can do it, but I move slowly and am concerned I might fall.
- ☐ I usually don't have to move sideways, so it's not an issue.

Is there a noticeable lag between the time when you rise up from a chair and when you are able to start walking?

- ☐ Yes
- ☐ No

Can you bend over at the waist and pick something up off the floor without discomfort or loss of balance?

- ☐ Yes
- ☐ No

Do you have low back pain that restricts your ability to bend at the waist?

- ☐ Yes
- ☐ No

Is your movement restricted by pain or limited range of motion in other joints?

- ☐ Yes
- ☐ No

Chapter 6). It's true that if we don't use it, we lose it, and that definitely applies to balance, flexibility, and agility.

As you reflect on your self-assessment, think about the movements and activities that currently restrict or impede your daily life. Keep in mind that your balance, flexibility, and agility can be improved, just as your cardiovascular fitness, strength, and muscle mass can be improved. Of course, if your movements are restricted because of osteoarthritis or injury, those conditions require medical attention before you attempt a rehab or exercise program.

Aging and Balance, Flexibility, and Agility

Eric is a 53-year-old married father of three (ages 23, 20, and 16) who has had an office job all of his professional life. Not surprisingly, Eric's health and fitness took a backseat to keeping up with the kids and their activities, chores around the house, and working full days. He hasn't slept well for years and has been gaining weight over time. He's also noticed that with weight gain and age has come a loss of agility and flexibility, so occasional pickup basketball games with friends have become a thing of the past. He tries to walk on his home treadmill at least 3 days a week and throws in some sit-ups, push-ups, and free weights when he's motivated and can spare the time. He recently injured his lower back when he bent over to grab a television remote control from under a chair, and occasional flare-ups of that nagging injury have further limited his ability to stay physically active. Eric feels as though he's fighting a losing battle but wants to work on things now that two of his three kids are out of the house and he has a little extra time for himself. Like many adults, Eric is overwhelmed by the seemingly impossible task of getting back into shape. He hardly knows where to start. Eric's best course is to continue his walking routine and calisthenics, gradually adding more days, more distance, more speed, and more reps as he begins to get into better shape. It will be easy for Eric to add a few flexibility, balance, and agility exercises to his routine so if he wants to get back to playing basketball, he'll be able to make that transition with less risk of injury and pain.

Most people sense the gradual decline in balance, agility, and flexibility that comes as we age and is made worse by a sedentary lifestyle, but few people appreciate that the long-term impact of that decline will threaten their ability to live independently. In fact, roughly 20% of those over 65 require help with at least one daily task, and 30% of people 60 years and older will fall within the next 6 months. Eric certainly isn't alone in his frustration over his inability to find the right physical activity plan to fit into a hectic lifestyle before things get so out of control that they will be extremely difficult to correct.

The US Department of Health and Human Services has a program called Healthy People 2020. One of the goals of this program is to reduce the frequency of falls among older adults because of the enormous health care costs associated with fall-related hospitalizations and rehabilitation, not to mention the impact that those injuries have on overall quality of life. In addition to lowering the frequency of falls, Healthy People 2020 hopes to reduce the risk of early death, coronary heart disease, stroke, high blood pressure, type 2 diabetes, breast and colon cancer, and depression. Not surprisingly, regular physical activity is an important part of Healthy People 2020 because of the well-established benefits of exercise for each of those maladies.

Equally unsurprising is that injuries, arthritis, and muscle weakness that affect the ankle, knee, and hip joints contribute to loss of balance, flexibility, and agility and can lead to chronic instability in the affected joints, increasing the risk of falling. How often have you heard stories about an otherwise healthy older person falling, breaking his or her leg or pelvis, and then never getting out of an assisted-living facility or dying soon after the injury? Falls are often devastating events for older adults, which is the main reason why maintaining balance, flexibility, and agility is absolutely essential to healthy aging.

Muscle weakness commonly occurs first in the lower limbs of older adults, likely because the legs are used less than the arms over time. Muscle weakness in the legs contributes to instability and overall decreased functional ability as we age. Regular physical activity can slow that decline and can, in some cases, even reverse the decline, lowering the risk of falling. In Chapter 6, we covered the numerous benefits of strength training; this chapter is a reminder that you can't neglect the characteristics—balance, flexibility, and agility—that will enable you to take full advantage of improved strength and cardiovascular fitness.

Clarifying the Science on Balance, Flexibility, and Agility

What Do Balance, Flexibility, and Agility Really Mean?

Even though these terms seem self-explanatory, it will be helpful to clarify how each attribute contributes to your continued ability to live independently and stay engaged in family and community activities. For the purposes of this chapter, we'll define *balance* as the ability to remain upright and steady. Your ability to balance relies on complex interactions among the information gathered by your eyesight; the balance mechanisms in your inner ears; and constant feedback from muscles, joints, and other body parts to your brain and spine. As you age, your balance is particularly important in avoiding falls and related injuries. *Flexibility* is the ability to bend and stretch easily without restriction or pain. Being flexible helps reduce the risk of injury associated with activities of daily life, such as bending over to pick something off the floor or twisting to reach into the back seat of a car to grab something. *Agility* refers to your capacity to change directions easily, quickly, and accurately, as we sometimes need to do to avoid falling over grandchildren, their toys, or your pets.

Why Are Balance, Flexibility, and Agility So Important?

Maintaining balance, flexibility, and agility as you age helps you stay active—and, in turn, this helps improve quality of life by reducing the risk of falling and other musculoskeletal injuries, such as low back pain and assorted joint injuries. You have probably experienced how difficult it can be to simply get dressed in the morning if back pain has flared up or if you've had a recent injury of almost any sort. Your younger self may have taken for granted the ability to perform everyday activities, such as getting dressed and undressed, moving in and out of a shower or bathtub, climbing stairs; reaching for something on a shelf; rising from a chair and walking quickly, and hopping out of the way of an unexpected obstacle. But with age, these mundane-yet-essential movements can become compromised as balance, flexibility, and agility slowly deteriorate—especially if you are overweight and out of shape.

Factors that Influence Balance, Flexibility, and Agility

As we age, there is a decline in the number of active sensory and motor nerves (neurons). Sensory nerves are responsible for providing feedback from muscles and joints to the spinal cord and brain to control posture, maintain balance, and constantly monitor where our arms and legs are positioned. All of this nerve activity occurs subconsciously to ensure that every movement of the body happens smoothly and successfully. Motor nerves enable conscious movements by stimulating muscles to contract and controlling the constant adjustments required to maintain posture and balance. As a result of the combination of growing older and being less physically active, sensory and motor nerve function slowly deteriorates, and so does balance and agility.

Our ability to remain balanced, particularly while we're walking, requires a combination of leg strength, joint stability, and balance, all controlled by unceasing sensory and motor nerve adjustments. Scientific research has taught us that muscle strength and cardiovascular fitness are independent entities; in other words, being strong doesn't mean that a person is aerobically fit, and vice versa. The same is true of balance, flexibility, and agility. Becoming stronger and more aerobically fit is no guarantee that your balance, flexibility, and agility will improve. In fact, we know these attributes are independent from one another and must be tested and trained separately. We have to pay attention to the entire package and make sure that our weekly physical activity includes strength, cardiovascular fitness, balance, flexibility, and agility training.

For those suffering from Alzheimer's disease, multiple sclerosis, or other neuromuscular disorders, studies show that regular physical activity improves the performance of daily tasks, along with enhanced cardiovascular fitness, flexibility, agility, balance, strength, and improvements in some mental functions, such as attention and memory. Improved balance, flexibility, and agility can go a long way to help people cope with the challenges of neuromuscular disorders.

Confronting Myths About Balance, Flexibility, and Agility

MYTH: Balance can't be improved.

REALITY: Just as agility and flexibility can be improved with proper training, so can balance. Although you might not be able to fully restore your balance to what it was when you walked across logs as a child, you should regularly practice balance exercises—standing on one foot with eyes closed is a good one—to help improve and maintain your ability to stay balanced. See the Useful Resources section on page 195 for websites that teach balance exercises.

MYTH: Too much stretching can actually make muscles weak.

REALITY: Not so—at least not in the most practical sense. Some research shows that strength is temporarily decreased immediately after muscles are stretched, a predictable response based on how the body is wired. However, that reduction in strength disappears after a few minutes.

MYTH: Stretching after exercise is the best time to improve flexibility.

REALITY: There is no ideal time to stretch. The best time to stretch is whenever you can fit it into your schedule. For some people, that may be after exercise, when they feel warm and limber. For others, stretching may be something to fit in while watching television or right before bedtime.

MYTH: You have to hold each stretch for at least 60 seconds to get any benefit.

REALITY: There are a variety of ways to stretch a muscle and increase its flexibility, but none of them require holding the stretch for longer than 15 to 30 seconds. Holding a stretch is sometimes referred to as static stretching. Other types of flexibility exercises involve movements—small and large. For example, dynamic stretching involves moving an extended limb throughout a range of motion, such as swinging one extended leg in a wide arc in front of the body. Other types of stretching include contractions of the stretched muscle or the opposing (contralateral; antagonistic) muscle immediately prior to a stretch to help facilitate greater flexibility. See the Useful Resources section on page 195 for websites that teach stretching exercises.

MYTH: Agility can't be improved after age 30.

REALITY: There's no doubt that agility deteriorates with age, especially after age 50, in large part because people stop doing activities that require changing directions quickly and accurately. But agility can be improved and its deterioration slowed by doing agility drills and exercises on a weekly basis. See the Useful Resources section on page 195 for websites that teach agility exercises.

MYTH: Stretching a muscle increases its length.

REALITY: Muscle length does not increase as flexibility improves, but its pliability does. Stretching makes muscles looser by regularly reminding the nervous system to slightly reduce its resting input to muscle cells. Even muscles at complete rest receive constant input from motor nerves that help maintain muscle tone so that when we decide to move—to rise from a chair, for example—there is no lag time before muscles contract sufficiently to produce the desired movement. Keep in mind that flexibility is also influenced by tendons, joint structures, and the sheaths of connective tissue that surround muscles (muscle fascia), so being flexible in the shoulder joints does not mean a person will be similarly flexible in other joints. With tendons and ligaments, the goal is not to stretch their length but to cause changes in their protein components, which improve elasticity. In muscles, stretching is thought to improve the elasticity of a large, spring-like protein called titin. Normal stretching exercises can accomplish all of those changes if done on a regular basis.

MYTH: Only stretches that cause some muscle pain are beneficial.

REALITY: Although one person's discomfort is another person's pain, there is no need for pain to improve flexibility. Stretching to the point where further motion is restricted, holding that position for 15 to 30 seconds, and repeating that stretch three or four times is sufficient to quickly improve flexibility.

Commonly Asked Questions About Balance, Flexibility, and Agility

Are the snap, crackle, and pop noises that sometimes occur during stretching and other activities signs that you might injure yourself?

The sounds and sensation we experience whenever we move, and especially when we stretch, are most often connective tissue (tendons and ligaments) moving across nearby bony structures. If these sounds are associated with pain, discomfort, or swelling, immediately stop and seek the advice or your physician or physical therapist. Otherwise, you can expect those sounds and sensations to disappear or at least become less annoying as you get into better shape.

Does stretching prevent injury?

Maybe, maybe not. Research is unclear as to the value of stretching for injury prevention. However, there is no good evidence that proper stretching increases injury risk, so if you feel that stretching helps you prevent injury, by all means continue.

What can be done to improve agility?

As we previously discussed, agility gradually deteriorates with age. After age 50, activities that require you to rapidly change direction wane. Howevere, this decline in agility can be slowed and even improved with regular physical activity, practice with agility drills, and participating in sports that require quick changes in direction. There are many ways to enhance your ability to change direction quickly and accurately. As a child, you might have played hopscotch, tag, and other games that honed your agility. The same might have been true with team sports or individual sports, such as tennis and racquetball. The internet is full of videos and other instructions for agility drills. These exercises are often targeted at athletes but can be easily modified to suit your needs.

Having the Confidence to Make a Plan Work for You

Many millions of Americans haven't exercised regularly for many decades; for them, beginning an exercise program is a daunting prospect. Beginning a commitment to regular physical activity can be made easier by starting with activities that emphasize balance, flexibility, and agility over aerobic fitness or strength training. Activities such as yoga, Zumba, Jazzercise, aerobic dance, novice-level Pilates, tai chi, dancing, and novice-level Body Pump, along with sports such as volleyball, softball, basketball, tennis, handball, pickleball, and soccer, are fun ways to improve balance, flexibility, and agility, with enhanced cardiovascular fitness and strength as added benefits as skills improve.

For those fitness enthusiasts who have spent decades moving in a straight line—runners, cyclists, swimmers, rowers—moving in other directions quickly and accurately can be a real challenge, which is all the more reason to include flexibility, balance, and agility exercises in your daily routine, perhaps during those occasions when you're watching television. Ideally, a qualified personal trainer, physical therapist, or certified athletic trainer can provide you with instruction and oversight that will rapidly improve your balance, flexibility, and agility and leave you with a number of different drills to do at home.

Conversation with an Expert

Dixie Stanforth, PhD, is a senior lecturer in the Department of Kinesiology and Health Education at the University of Texas, Austin. Dixie teaches students how to maintain a healthy lifestyle and actually practices what she preaches. She knows adding flexibility and agility training is just as important as doing cardio and strength training. Her motivation? She says,

> A lot of what I do for exercise is to keep me in shape to hike the "14ers" [14,000-foot mountains] in Colorado in the summertime. I still remember the first yoga class I took about 15 years ago, and my response was that I was really bad at it—and so I needed to do it! I wasn't as stable or balanced as I thought I was, and I definitely needed to add a flexibility component to my workouts. I try to be aware of and willing to have a growth mindset so that I move toward something that is challenging, rather than avoiding it.

Dixie and her husband, Phil, have hiked 27 different 14ers, and several of them more than once.

> Dixie tries to be active every day, explaining: I am fortunate in that I love to move, and being physically active is as much a part of my life as brushing my teeth! I mix up the intensity of my workouts so I have recovery days, but I do some type of physical activity pretty much every day."

Her daily workouts have another benefit aside from the physical; she also values the mental power that comes with exercise. She adds:

> I do my best thinking during a workout. I also do some training with friends, so that's a chance to catch up and stay connected. And I love to eat, so regular exercise is a way to ensure that I can eat all the foods I enjoy.

For Dixie, living with celiac disease means eating gluten free, and an allergy to the protein casein, found in dairy foods, adds another layer of restriction to Dixie's food choices. But because of the restrictions, she "eats a lot of fresh, whole foods and very few packaged foods that might have gluten or casein in the ingredient list." Her favorite treat is dark chocolate "in pretty much any form!"

As Dixie is in her mid-50s, she does think about her family history of cancer and other chronic diseases but says, "I try to not be anxious about my genetics; I eat well, exercise regularly, and basically do all I can to stay healthy." Her philosophy is one we agree with: "Find things you love to do and foods you love to eat, and do/eat them regularly."

How the Authors Improve and Maintain Balance, Flexibility, and Agility

Chris: After hip replacement surgery at age 62, I knew I had to do more than physical therapy to improve my balance, flexibility, and agility. In the years leading up to the surgery, my exercise was restricted to walking, and because I developed a limp, my back also hurt. (When I told my orthopedist that my back hurt, he said, "That is just because your hip is pissing off your back.") In other words, while compensating for a bad hip joint, I altered my body position and gait, which led to other problems. After surgery, my solution was to take a 60-minute yoga class at my local YMCA twice a week. The class spends equal amount of time on yoga poses, balance work, and stretching. I recently told the instructor that her class had improved the quality of my life. I no longer feel minor aches and pains during routine activities. My balance is greatly improved, and I can put my hands flat on the ground without bending my knees. I'm not sure I could have done that when I was 20. The other benefit of yoga is that it is one of the few times where my mind is not racing at 100 mph. I find it relaxing and renewing for body and mind.

Bob: On a snowy night in late January 2016, I broke my left ankle when I lost control of my fat-tire mountain bike while trying to cross an icy patch on a local bike trail. Fortunately, no surgery, pins, or plates were needed; compression wrap, frequent icing, six weeks in a stabilization boot, and lots of rehab exercise took care of most of the healing. I can now walk, jog, cycle, and swim without restriction, even though the ankle remains a little swollen and occasionally sore a year later. I'm still working on improving the ankle's range of motion and regaining strength, mobility, and especially balance.

Standing just on that foot is a wobbly and short-lived experience, an indication that I need to do more balance exercises to regain normal function. I don't want that ankle to restrict my lifestyle—it occasionally trips me up while working in the yard—or increase the risk of falls as I age, so improving my balance is important and something for me to work on in the months and years ahead.

Useful Resources

Centers for Disease Control and Prevention (www.cdc.gov/mmwr/volumes/65/wr/mm6536a3.htm)

▷ *Summary of the risks of physical inactivity among adults aged 50 years and older, and how communities can address this*

Centers for Disease Control and Prevention (www.cdc.gov/steadi/pdf/tug_test-a.pdf)

▷ *Instructions for a simple Timed Up-and-Go test that health professionals may use to assess the risk of falls in older adults*

Fitness Blender (www.fitnessblender.com)

▷ *Example of an online and app-based fitness program; search this site for sessions that focus on whole-body flexibility*

Go4Life from the National Institute on Aging (https://go4life.nia.nih.gov/tip-sheets/exercise-improve-your-balance)

▷ *Step-by-step instructions and illustrations for simple exercises to do at home to improve balance, flexibility, and agility*

SECTION 3

BE WELL

IN THEORY, IF you eat well and move well, you will be well, but there is more to it than that. In this section, we cover several topics that help us be well; not all of them are food or fitness related. However, there is one food and fitness topic that most adults care very much about as they age: weight management. We don't encourage dieting in the traditional sense of quick weight loss, which is typically followed by weight gain. Instead, we encourage adoption of healthy eating patterns with an emphasis on consuming right-sized portions, eating mindfully, and realizing that a healthy body isn't determined by a number on the scale. Aging brings changes to your body composition, and it is unlikely you will ever look like you did in your 20s when you are age 60 or beyond, but good health is not beyond your control.

We also know that sleep, stress, and social support all influence optimal aging. Getting good-quality sleep, seeking ways to be resilient in the face of stress, and strengthening our social connections can impact our feelings about aging and, in indirect ways, help us with our food and fitness goals. Emerging research suggests that sleep deprivation alters hormones that encourage body fat storage, and most everyone has experienced stress eating. Our friends and family can help us with fitness by becoming exercise buddies to encourage and hold us accountable to a commitment to be active.

We conclude this section with the harsh reality that bad things can and do happen as we age. It is natural to worry about future health for ourselves and our loved ones as we age. Aging is a risk factor for many of the most common chronic diseases: high blood pressure, heart disease, stroke, arthritis, and cancer. Once disease or injury strikes, you can't turn back time and dwell on what you might have done differently, which is a very common reaction. You can only move forward to be the healthiest you can be while living with chronic disease and recovering from or adapting to injuries. Embrace the new reality, and find new ways to be physically active and eat healthy.

CHAPTER

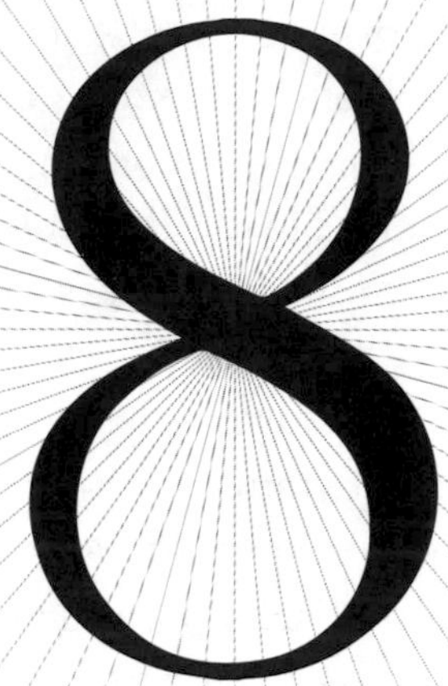

WEIGHT MANAGEMENT AFTER 50

The Bottom Line

Managing body weight is a top concern for many aging adults. Physiological changes contribute to altering our body composition as we age, but those changes are accelerated by an environment that encourages overeating and a sedentary lifestyle. We can halt some of the changes through sensible food choices, regular aerobic exercise, and strength training. Following are some key points to keep in mind for managing your weight after age 50.

- Two easy self-assessments are recommended to learn your risk of developing chronic disease. First, determine your body mass index (BMI) using accurate height and weight measurements and aim for a healthy weight range. Second, measure your waist circumference to determine if you have too much belly fat.
- Set health goals, not weight goals; weight loss or maintenance often follows when you achieve such goals as lowering blood pressure or improving strength and aerobic fitness.

- **If your BMI and waist circumference are in the high range, focus on eating and exercise for health to support weight loss. Losing just 5% of your body weight as a target can reap big health benefits.**
- **Give up the cycle of searching for the best diet and setting unrealistic weight-loss goals. You *can* be too thin, and seeking skinny is not healthy as you age.**
- **Learn to estimate portion sizes and make an effort to right-size portions at home and when dining out.**
- **Monitor your weight frequently to avoid gaining a couple of pounds every year.**
- **Identify with the habits of successful losers: reduce screen time, exercise daily, eat breakfast, and monitor your weight.**

ASSESS YOURSELF: IN REVIEW

Take the Assess Yourself quiz on the next page before reading on.

The key to managing your weight is first to get an accurate assessment of your weight. We will show you a simple way to assess your weight and get you on the right path. We believe everyone should have an accurate digital scale, one that you can calibrate to keep it accurate. By having a scale and using it frequently, you won't be surprised when your doctor weighs you. You won't have to mutter that the doctor's scale must be inaccurate because you will know your usual weight range. We will show you how to calculate your BMI from accurate height and weight measurements and explain what your BMI really tells you. This is also a good time to take stock of your history with weight-loss diets. If you followed a weight-loss plan and were able to keep most of the weight off, congratulations. However, there are many adults who are always either on or just coming off a diet. We'll show you that there isn't a single best diet for weight loss and reveal some strategies to help you maintain your weight. We also included alcohol in this chapter because many of us don't think about the extra calories that a glass or two (or three) of wine or beer contains and how that can contribute to extra pounds.

Assess Yourself: Managing Your Weight

Do you have a reliable scale?
- ☐ Yes
- ☐ No

If yes, how do you know it's reliable?

____

How often do you weigh yourself?
- ☐ Daily
- ☐ Weekly
- ☐ Monthly
- ☐ Periodically
- ☐ Never

How do you feel when you see the numbers on the scale?

____

Compared with when you were 25 years old, do you weigh:
- ☐ The same
- ☐ More
- ☐ Less

Do you know your BMI?
- ☐ Yes
- ☐ No

Do you know how to interpret BMI?
- ☐ Yes
- ☐ No

What is your waist size?

____

Have you ever been on a weight-loss diet?
- ☐ Yes
- ☐ No

If yes, which one(s)?

____

Did you lose weight on the diet?
- ☐ Yes
- ☐ No

If yes, how much, and how long did you keep the weight off?

____

What do you think is a healthy weight for you?

____

Do you consume alcohol?
- ☐ Yes
- ☐ No

If yes, do you drink beer, wine, or spirits?

____

How much alcohol do you consume daily?

____

How much alcohol do you consume weekly?

____

How has the amount of alcohol you consume changed as you have gotten older?
- ☐ Increased
- ☐ Same
- ☐ Decreased

Introduction

Randall has a love/hate relationship with quick weight-loss diets. In college, he was a two-sport athlete (football and track) and kept his 6-foot 3-inch frame at 200 pounds. At that weight, his BMI was 25, and he had much more muscle than fat. He believed he would always stay active—the habits of training and competition were "in his blood"—but then life happened. After college, his regional sales manager job kept him on the road 4 or 5 days a week. He got married and raised a family and jokes that he gained weight with each of his wife's pregnancies and never lost the baby weight. Today, at 67, Randall weighs 290 pounds and is worried that he will hit the 300-pound mark soon if he doesn't take control. When the high-fat, low-carbohydrate diet craze was popular, Randall became an Atkins addict and lost 35 pounds the first time he went on the diet. Unfortunately, he gained back 40 pounds when he went off the diet. He has tried the no-carb approach six times over the past 20 years—always losing a significant number of pounds, but always gaining it back, usually with a few pounds more than his starting weight. Randall loved the thrill of rapid weight loss, but after 3 or 4 weeks on a diet, he began to get headaches and had no energy. He still works in sales, but most of his days are spent in an office, behind a computer terminal, and he entertains clients by taking them out to lunch and dinner about 4 days a week. Today, he is contemplating intermittent fasting as a way to lose weight and keep it off.

Does our biology conspire against us to cause gain weight as we age or is it our lifestyles that make it harder to keep the pounds in check? Most likely, it's a little of both. Randall's story illustrates what happens to many adults as they age. His sports participation dropped off when he started working and raising a family. A sedentary job and frequent dining out upset the energy balance equation: less calories out and more calories in led to gradual weight gain.

It's important to understand how some physiological changes make it harder to maintain weight as the years go by:

- Basal metabolic rate (BMR) is the biggest contributor to how many calories are burned every day. BMR is the number of calories needed each day for life-sustaining processes, like breathing, keeping your heart beating, and repairing your body's tissues. BMR declines about 2% per decade, starting at about the age of 25. However, some of that decline is related to loss of lean body mass. Much of that age-related decline can be reverted by preserving and building your muscles, as we discussed in Chapter 6.

- Hormonal changes, especially for women around the time of menopause, contribute to changing body composition. Decreasing levels of estrogen contribute to loss of bone mass and increased storage of fat inside the abdomen. Intra-abdominal fat is called visceral fat by medical professionals and belly fat by the rest of us. In general, women tend to be pear-shaped, but after menopause, many women find they are carrying more belly fat. Women also burn slightly less energy (fewer calories) when they no longer have monthly menstrual cycles.
- Men also experience some changes in hormone levels that contribute to weight gain and changes in body composition, but the changes are not as dramatic as the loss of estrogen in women. Men experience a decrease in secretion of growth hormone, with peak loss occurring around age 70. Decreasing levels of growth hormone can result in decreased muscle mass and increased body fat storage. Men tend to be more apple shaped, carrying extra fat inside the abdomen. Belly fat is more likely to contribute to a constellation of symptoms called metabolic syndrome, which, if unchecked, can lead to high blood pressure, heart disease, and diabetes. Decreasing growth hormone further accelerates storage of belly fat.

APPLE- AND PEAR-SHAPED BODY TYPES

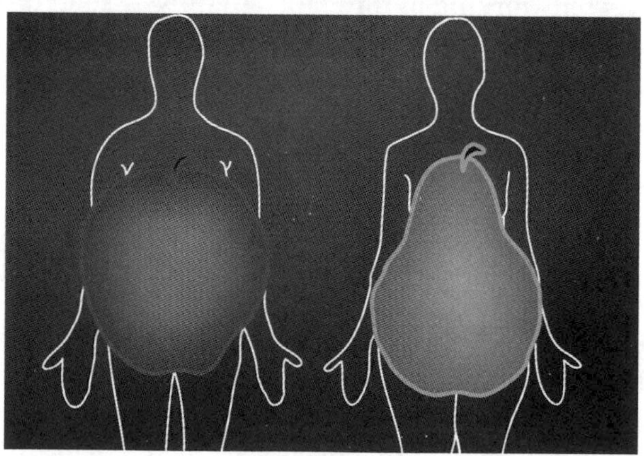

Although aging is unavoidable and does present challenges with maintaining muscle mass and losing body fat, lifestyle also plays a major role in the ability to achieve and maintain a healthy weight. Of course, this includes both food and fitness. When it comes to our food choices, humans are genetically programmed to like sweets and fats and to store body fat for lean times. Fortunately, most of us never experience lean times, so our storage deposits of fat continue to grow. A more significant concern is that portion sizes have increased over the past several decades, and we are encouraged to eat for recreation and emotional comfort. The table on page 204 shows a few examples of how increasing portion sizes lead to more calories consumed. As food has become more affordable, we now think of large portions as normal when, in fact, they are larger than we need. To top it off, food is everywhere; no longer confined to grocery stores or restaurants, food is within easy reach 24/7.

Another concern is that modern conveniences have eroded the calorie-burning activities our parents performed every day, and even though these activities seem minor, they can add up to burning many calories throughout the day. Consider just a few of the changes from one generation to the next:

- Drive-through access to banking, dry cleaning, pharmacies, fast food, and even our morning coffee have reduced the need to get out of our cars and walk.
- Cars have automatic transmissions, power windows, keyless entry, push-button starters, and a remote opener for the garage, so there's no need to actively engage in these tasks. Driverless cars are on the horizon, further eroding the need to expend energy.
- Pay-at-the pump gas means not having to walk the few steps to the station store to pay for fuel.
- In the home, we have little to do for most housecleaning chores besides loading the dishwasher or washer and dryer and pushing a button to start; many of us remember our parents hanging the wash on a clothesline or scrubbing dishes at the kitchen sink. Devices such as robot vacuum cleaners and electronic

PORTION SIZES: 30 YEARS AGO VS TODAY

	Serving Size		Calorie Count	
	30 Years Ago	***Today***	***25 Years Ago***	***Today***
Muffin	1.5 oz	5 oz	210	500
Bagel	3-inch diameter	6-inch diameter	140	350
French Fries	2.4 oz	6.9 oz	210	610
Pepperoni Pizza	2 slices	2 slices	500	850
Cheesecake	3 oz	7 oz	260	640
Chicken Caesar Salad	1.5 cups	3.5 cups	390	790
Movie-Theater Popcorn	Small (5 cups)	Large (11 cups)	270	630
Fast-Food Meal	Burger, fries, and soft drink	Quarter-pound burger, large fries, and soft drink	590	1,200

desktop assistants can perform many household chores via hands-free, voice-activated commands.

- Screen time has increased. More time is spent using computers, tablets, and cell phones and binge-watching big-screen televisions. And if you want to remind your grandchildren how old you are, just tell them about the time when you had to get up from the couch to change the television channel.
- Remember when you had to move to answer a ringing telephone? Now, it is likely that your phone is never out of reach, so there's no need to move to communicate with someone.

Changes in body composition and weight may be inevitable as we age, but we can take control of these changes through our food choices and exercise habits. Increasing body weight sets the stage for chronic diseases like high blood pressure, heart disease, type 2 diabetes, gallstones, sleep apnea, respiratory problems, and even some

Factors that Influence Weight Gain, Loss, or Maintenance

Resting metabolic rate (RMR): the energy or calories needed for everyday life

Physical activity energy expenditure: the energy or calories expended by planned activities

Thermic effect of food: the energy or calories needed for digestion and absorption of food

Nonexercise activity thermogenesis (NEAT): the energy or calories expended in fidgeting-type behaviors

Energy efficiency: the body's efficiency at extracting energy from food and/or storing it as fat

Energy (calorie) intake

Age

Gender

Response to food cues

Stress (emotional eating)

Medications (many prescription drugs can contribute to weight gain; see the Useful Resources section on page 227 for suggested reading about drugs that can influence weight gain)

Sleep

Genetics

Diet composition

Overestimating physical activity energy expenditure (and eating more as a result)

More sitting, less moving on exercise days

Sensitivity to hunger and satiety hormones

cancers. The good news is that losing just 5% of your body weight, a 7.5-pound weight loss for a 152-pound person, results in many positive health benefits and lowers the risk for many health conditions. So starting small and setting health goals (eg, lowering blood pressure, lowering blood sugar, improving aerobic conditioning and strength) can have positive, long-term benefits.

Clarifying the Science on Weight Management

Just as there is no best diet, there is no one factor that contributes to weight gain or loss. Genetics, as well as social and behavioral factors, all play a role. The Obesity Society says that more than 60 factors can impact energy balance and body weight. Just a few of these are listed in the box on page 205. These factors, combined with the fact that energy balance is more complex than the simple energy in equals energy out equation, mean that there is no one weight loss, gain, or maintenance plan that works for everyone. Let's take a look at what is known about weight management.

Understanding the Concept of a Healthy Body Weight

A healthy body weight is one that decreases your risk of developing chronic diseases. Body weight is used as a surrogate measure for health only because it is easy, not because it tells us everything important about body composition. A common measure used to classify underweight, normal weight, overweight, and obesity is BMI, or body mass index, which shows the relationship between height and weight and is used to assess the risk of developing disease. There are four BMI categories:

< 18.5 = underweight

18.5 to 24.99 = healthy weight

25 to 30 = overweight

> 30 = obese

BMI values were developed by studying large groups of people and diseases common in these populations. Since there is great variation in body shape and size, a range was created to classify a healthy weight. How do you measure your BMI? It only requires knowing your height and weight, which may sound easy, but research shows that people tend to overestimate height and underestimate weight. Once you have accurate measures of your height and weight, plug them into an online calculator, such as the one at the National Heart, Lung, and Blood Institute website (see the Useful Resources section on page 227). You can also use the table below to find a healthy weight range for your height based on BMI tables. Notice that there is a fairly wide range of body weights classified as healthy for each height, which accounts for varying body shapes and sizes. Remember that BMI is used to assess risk for disease, not appearance. There is increased disease risk with a BMI that is either too low or too high.

HEALTHY WEIGHT RANGE BY HEIGHT

Height	Healthy Weight Range in Pounds*
5 feet 0 inches	95–126
5 feet 1 inches	98–130
5 feet 2 inches	100–133
5 feet 3 inches	104–138
5 feet 4 inches	107–145
5 feet 5 inches	111–149
5 feet 6 inches	114–153
5 feet 7 inches	118–159
5 feet 8 inches	122–164
5 feet 9 inches	125–168
5 feet 10 inches	128–173
5 feet 11 inches	132–178
6 feet 0 inches	136–183
6 feet 1 inches	140–189
6 feet 2 inches	144–194
6 feet 3 inches	147–199

*Based on a BMI of 18.5 to 24.99

Adapted from Body Mass Index Table, National Heart, Lung, and Blood Institute

In addition to knowing your BMI, we recommend two other tools that can help you assess your body weight and determine if changes need to be made: an old-fashioned cloth tape measure and an accurate bathroom scale.

First, measure your height by standing barefoot with your heels against the wall (preferably a wall without a baseboard on a floor without carpet). Stand tall and have someone mark the wall at the top of your head (use a book or other flat surface held flat on your head, and compress your hair if necessary). Use the tape measure against the wall to find your true height.

Then, weigh yourself on a digital bathroom scale. Do this first thing in the morning while wearing minimal clothing, after urinating and before you eat. Plug your height and weight into an online calculator to get your BMI.

BMI is moderately related to body fatness, but it is not an assessment for body fat. An athlete, for example, may have a high BMI and have little fat but a whole lot of muscle. Conversely, an older adult might have a healthy BMI but at the same time may have lost muscle with a gradual increase in body fat. Researchers call that sarcopenic obesity. So we recommend measuring waist circumference, which is a good surrogate marker for belly fat.

- Standing tall, measure your middle, just above your hip bones and below your belly button. Take a deep breath, let it out, and then measure your waist in inches.
- For men, if your waist is 40 inches or greater and for women, if it is 35 inches or greater, you are storing more visceral, or belly, fat than is recommended for good health. (Waist circumference values for Asian men and women are slightly lower than these values; for guidelines for different ethnicities, see the Useful Resources section on page 227.)

As mentioned earlier, men tend to store extra fat in the belly (apple shape), and women store it in their thighs and hips (pear shape), but around age 50, hormonal changes in women can direct fat storage to their bellies. In both men and women, fat stored in the belly can secrete hormones that disrupt the way the body handles blood sugar, increasing the risk for type 2 diabetes and heart disease. Despite claims to the contrary, there are no magic foods that burn belly fat, but aerobic activity and calorie reduction can certainly help. You can do crunches all day, but you won't have a six pack unless you lose a significant amount of body fat. We don't think having a six pack is a worthy goal for most people, but neither is having a belly that looks like a basketball. As discussed in earlier chapters, spot reduction doesn't work; some people will always store some extra fat in the belly or hips. The key is not to let the fat deposits continue to grow unchecked. That is why an assessment of both your BMI and your waist circumference gives some baseline information to set a course to improve health and decrease the risk of disease.

Pros and Cons of Body-Fat Testing

Since BMI doesn't reveal the amount of body fat you carry, should you get your body fat tested? To get the most accurate body fat percentage, researchers rely on a sophisticated measurement technique that uses expensive equipment, but that type of testing is out of reach for most people. Athletes often have access to these fancy methods, like air-displacement plethysmography, which involves sitting in a chamber called the BOD POD to assess body fat. But for most adults, less expensive, and somewhat less accurate, methods are used, such as skinfold thickness, which uses calipers to pinch fat in various places around the body, or bioelectrical impedance analysis, which uses a handheld or standing device. These techniques are often used in gyms by personal trainers or at health fairs for a quick assessment. While these assessments can give an estimate of body fat, results are highly variable. The person doing the measurement is one source of error. Training is needed to use the equipment and to conduct the measurement. The error rate for body fat measurements can be 10% under the best circumstances and as high as 15% to 20% for the type of assessment done in a gym or at a health fair.

While you might be tempted to rely on these less accurate ways to measure body fat, we recommend that you start with your BMI and waist circumference and use those numbers to determine if change is needed. If you want to assess your body fat level, be mindful of the limitations. Body fat testing is best done as a serial measurement to assess change over time; a one-time measurement does little to provide information about your health.

Do Your Calories In Equal Your Calories Out?

You may have read that managing your weight is a simple matter of balancing how many calories you consume each day with how many calories you burn during normal activities, plus exercise. This may sound logical and easy, but the reality is more complex. First, how do you know how many calories you need every day? While we don't advocate counting calories, here are some general estimates of how many daily calories 50+ men and women need, depending on their activity level:

- A sedentary woman needs about 1,600 calories, and a sedentary man needs about 2,000 calories.
- A moderately active woman needs about 1,800 calories, and a moderately active man needs about 2,200 to 2,400 calories.
- An active woman needs about 2,000 calories, and an active man needs about 2,400 to 2,800 calories.

Compare these calorie levels with that of a Tour de France cyclist who rides about 110 miles a day over rugged terrain. The cyclist needs more than 6,000 calories a day! Keep in mind that men generally need more calories than women because they have more lean muscle; that is why men can often eat more than women and not gain weight. It's not fair, we know, but that is the reality. Another consideration is that shorter people generally need fewer calories than taller people. All things being equal, a 4-foot 11-inch woman shouldn't eat as much as a 5-foot 10-inch woman. More body surface area (taller) means more calories burned.

When we were in school, we were taught that 1 pound of body fat stores 3,500 calories, but we now know that is an overly simplistic notion. To illustrate, cutting 500 calories a day for 7 days should result in a 1-pound weight loss, if that equation holds true. However, some people will lose more than 1 pound and some will lose less, depending on such factors as body composition, activity level, and more. When you restrict calories—and especially when you significantly reduce carbohydrate—the first things you lose are muscle stores of carbohydrate, called glycogen. Each unit of glycogen is stored with water, so when you first start dieting, you lose glycogen plus water weight. We think that is why people are so excited after the first week of dieting; there's a noticeable drop in the numbers on the scale. Then, after a few weeks, weight loss slows or even plateaus. This is your body's way of telling you that fewer calories are needed to maintain the lower body weight. To continue to lose weight, you have to further cut calories or increase your calorie-burning exercise. Again, we say, no fair, but the physiology of weight loss is complex. And to make things even harder, your hormones cope by telling the brain you are hungry.

You will also hear simple advice like, "Cutting 100 calories a day from your diet, the equivalent of one small apple, can result in a 10-pound weight loss in a year." That sounds easy, but after cutting calories at one meal, most people tend to compensate at the next meal by eating more calories. To lose weight and maintain that loss is no easy matter. That is why we suggest eating for health, not for external factors, like losing weight for a high-school reunion or for fitting into a smaller suit or dress for a family wedding. While external factors might be motivating in the short term, they rarely work in the long term. We suggest the following strategies for weight control among older adults:

- Accurately assess your weight and current risk for chronic diseases.
- Assess your current eating habits and compare them to one of the four plans presented in Chapter 2.
- Eat for health, and don't make weight loss the primary focus (unless prescribed by your doctor).
- Increase your physical activity by including both aerobic fitness and strength training.
- If you've been on and off diets most of your life, ditch the diet plans and first pledge to maintain your current weight and not gain weight. You can do this through self-monitoring with regular weigh-ins, along with food and exercise tracking.

Are All Calories Equal?

There's no simple answer to this question. We know that 1 gram of carbohydrate and 1 gram of protein each contain about 4 calories per gram, fat has about 9 calories per gram, and alcohol has about 7. These numbers might suggest that you should ditch the fat and alcohol to cut calories and eat more carbohydrate and protein. But the problem with that approach is that protein and fat are the nutrients most tied to satiety, or the feeling of fullness and satisfaction. One hundred calories of sugar cookies versus one hundred calories of peanuts may provide the body with the same amount of energy, but the peanuts will help keep you feeling full, while at the same time providing quality nutrients (eg, protein, vitamins, minerals, and fiber) not found in the cookies. That's why you should try to incorporate protein and healthy fats (for a list of healthy fats, see Chapter 2) in every meal and include high-fiber carbs, which also help fill you up. This doesn't mean you should give up carbs altogether and never eat a cookie, but when looking for a snack, make substitutions that will keep you satisfied. See the table below for some examples of simple substitutions to make over meals and snacks that will keep you feeling full and boost nutrient intake.

SIMPLE SUBSTITUTIONS

	If you eat this:	**Try this instead:**
Breakfast	*Coffee and doughnut*	Coffee with oatmeal and chopped walnuts
	Fruit juice	Whole fruit
	Three-egg ham omelet	Two-egg omelet with veggies
	Toast and jam	Whole grain toast with almond butter
Lunch	*Tuna salad sandwich*	Tuna salad lettuce wrap
	BLT with chips	Chicken and avocado in a pita pocket
	Burger and fries	Grilled fish tacos with guacamole
Dinner	*8-ounce ribeye*	4-ounce filet
	Loaded baked potato	Small baked potato with broccoli and cheese
	Fried onion rings	Grilled onions and peppers
Snacks	*Energy bar*	Handful of mixed nuts
	Milkshake	Smoothie made with Greek yogurt and berries
	Cookies	Fig bars

Do Any Diets Really Work for Weight Loss?

All diets work; by that we mean that you can lose weight on almost any reduced-calorie meal plan, as long as you stick to it. But just like Randall in our opening case study discovered most diets ultimately fail because they are restrictive and don't lead to real changes in eating habits. Because diet is a four-letter word and it starts with D-I-E, we prefer not to use it. Instead we advocate for healthy eating, an active life, enjoyment of foods, and not counting calories. The eating plans presented in Chapter 2 can all lead to weight loss and improved health simply by moderating portion sizes. However, we know some of you have questions about popular weight-loss diets, so we provide the premise, promises, pros, and pitfalls of some popular diets in the table on pages 214 and 215.

What We Know About Weight Loss and Maintenance from Successful Losers

In 2016, the media zeroed in on the reality television show *The Biggest Loser*—notably, on the fact that many participants regained their lost weight. While the methods of weight loss on this show are not realistic for most of us, the media reports distorted the truth. Of the 14 people who had appeared on the show and were followed up on for 6 years after the show ended, two weighed more than they did at the start of the show and three regained all of their lost weight, but eight kept at least half of the weight off, and one actually lost more weight. These results are similar to the trends seen with weight-loss diets and gastric reduction (bariatric) surgeries: some weight regain is likely, but the fact remains that losing even a small amount of weight and keeping it off has health benefits.

Since 1994, the National Weight Control Registry has collected data on individuals who have lost significant amounts of weight and kept it off. Among its participants, the average weight loss was 66 pounds, and the loss was maintained for more than 5 ½ years. About 45% of the participants lost weight on their own, while 55% used

POPULAR DIET PROMISES AND PITFALLS

Raw Foods Diet

Premise: Raw foods are healthier than cooked foods because cooking destroys most of the vitamins and minerals in foods and all of the phytonutrients (plant nutrients) in foods.

Promises: Weight loss, improved health, environmentally friendly

Pros:

- Diet is rich in fruits and vegetables.
- It eliminates processed foods with added sugar, salt, and fat.

Pitfalls:

- Meal preparation can be tedious, and it can be difficult to dine out
- Some nutrients are less available to the body in raw foods; cooking improves digestion and absorption of some nutrients.
- It advocates consuming raw milk, cheese, and meat, which can cause food-borne illnesses.

Gluten-Free Diet

Premise: Gluten, a protein in wheat, cannot be properly digested by many Americans and should be eliminated.

Promises: Weight loss, improved health

Pros:

- Gluten-free diets are necessary for the 3 million Americans with diagnosed celiac disease and one million more with gluten sensitivity unrelated to celiac disease. However, there is no evidence that people who do not have these conditions should avoid gluten.
- Eliminating gluten found in wheat, rye, barley, triticale, and spelt improves symptoms and health in those with celiac disease and non-celiac gluten sensitivity.
- Other grain foods can be included, such as rice, corn, spelt, quinoa, amaranth, millet, potatoes, buckwheat, tapioca, and wild rice.

Pitfalls:

- A gluten-free diet is not a recommended weight loss plan.
- Gluten-free packaged foods can be higher in fat, calories, and sugar than gluten-containing foods and may be more costly.

Paleo Diet

Premise: Modern life has ruined our food supply. Returning to the diet eaten by our distant ancestors will restore health and significantly reduce acute and chronic diseases.

Promises: Weight loss, improved health, and an eating plan better matched to our biology than the typical Western diet

Pros:

- Protein-rich foods on the diet (wild game and fish, grass-fed beef) are lower in saturated fat than most meats in a Western diet.
- It includes foods high in fiber, vitamins, and minerals and low in refined sugar, sodium, and fat.
- Overall, the diet plan could increase awareness of what foods are healthier than others.

Pitfalls:

- The diet eliminates dairy, grains, and legumes, and when entire food groups are eliminated, there is potential for nutrient shortfalls and a sense of deprivation.
- Eating more red meat is associated with increased risk of colon cancer.
- Despite claims to the contrary, no one is really sure what and how much Paleolithic people ate.

Intermittent Fasting Diet

Premise: Intermittent fasting can help achieve a weight loss of 1 or more pounds per week and reduces the risk of chronic diseases.

Promises: Weight loss, protection against cardiovascular diseases and cancer

Pros:

- Reducing calories two days a week (semi-fasting) to 500 calories for women and 600 calories for men could result in weight loss.
- It may be an easier way to diet for individuals who have a hard time with consistent portion control.
- It may increase awareness of how many calories are in foods and beverages.

Pitfalls:

- People who fast may unknowingly increase calorie consumption on nonfasting days.
- It could be hard to maintain high-intensity or long-duration exercise on fasting days.
- This diet is not recommended for people with diabetes.
- There is very limited research on this diet's long-term health benefit or harm.

Glycemic Index Diet

Premise: Some carbohydrate-containing foods have a high glycemic index, meaning that these foods affect your blood sugar levels more quickly compared with other carbohydrate foods, proteins, and fats. Technically, glycemic index is a measure of the effect of 50 grams of carbohydrate in a food on blood sugar levels.

Promises: Weight loss, stabilizes blood sugar to control diabetes, reduces risk of cardiovascular disease

Pros:

- Diets based on the glycemic index can help limit foods high in added sugar.
- Glycemic index can help dieters make healthier food choices.
- The diet does not eliminate entire foods groups, so is unlikely to lead to any nutrient shortfalls.

Pitfalls:

- The glycemic index is not known for every food, even within a category. For example, some types of ice cream have a higher glycemic index and some have a lower glycemic index depending on the ingredients used to make the it.
- Many factors influence the glycemic index ranking of foods, such as variety, ripeness, cooking method, and portion size. For example, carrots are listed as a high glycemic index food, but it takes 1½ pounds of carrots to provide 50 grams of carbohydrate.
- When foods are eaten together in a meal, the effect on blood sugar levels is different from when they are consumed as single foods.

some type of structured program. The successful losers had the following habits that helped keep them on track:

- 78% ate breakfast every day
- 75% weighed themselves at least once a week
- 62% watched less than 10 hours of television per week
- 90% exercised for 1 hour every day

The researchers concluded that many methods work to lose weight, but just as important are the habits that keep the weight off for long-term maintenance. No one size fits all when it comes to weight loss.

A Sensible Way to Gain Weight

Most adults we talk to want to lose or maintain weight, but this is a chapter on weight management, and some individuals want to *gain* weight. The best way to gain weight is to undertake a strength training program, as discussed in Chapter 6. Simple, at-home exercises that work all the major muscle groups will help develop muscle mass. An eating plan that emphasizes calorie-dense foods and eating frequency can augment strength training. If you would like to gain muscle mass, eat 5 or 6 times per day, and try these ideas:

- Spread nut or seed butters on toast, bread, or biscuits.
- Incorporate full-fat dairy foods.
- Break out the blender and make calorie-dense shakes or smoothies using protein powders, frozen fruit, and full-fat yogurt or milk.
- Replace water with full-fat milk when making cream soups or hot chocolate.
- Instant dry milk powder is an inexpensive protein powder that can boost calories and protein. It can be added to mashed potatoes, macaroni and cheese, cream soups, hot cereal, and even milk.

Confronting Myths About Weight Management

MYTH: Everyone has an ideal body weight.

REALITY: There is no such thing as an ideal weight. Your weight fluctuates a couple of pounds every day, usually related to hydration levels. A healthy weight range is a better description than ideal weight. Everyone comes in different shapes and sizes (tall and thin or short and stocky and everything in between), and there is no ideal weight that is right for everyone.

MYTH: You can't lose weight past the age of 50.

REALITY: Aging adults can and do lose weight with diet and exercise. It might be more challenging to lose weight as we age, but it's not impossible. We suggest setting health goals instead of weight goals; often, weight loss follows as a result of setting health goals, like lowering blood pressure or blood sugar or getting in better physical shape to participate in a community cycling event or run a 5K road race.

MYTH: You can never be too thin.

REALITY: We are sure you have heard that you can never be too rich or too thin, but being too thin has disadvantages that being too rich doesn't have. Being underweight can leave you with little body fat reserves to draw on in times of illness or infection, and carrying a healthy level of body fat affords some protection to bones. Therefore, a BMI below 18.5 is considered unhealthy.

MYTH: The latest diet is the greatest diet.

REALITY: Diet books are a multimillion-dollar industry. We've both reviewed our fair share of diet and exercise books over the past 30 years and agree with Malcolm Gladwell, best-selling author and journalist, who summed up diet books perfectly in a 1998 *New Yorker* article titled "The Pima Paradox" (the Useful Resources section on page 227 provides the link to his website and the article). He said every diet book is written the same way: they all start out with a sad personal story, followed by an "Aha!" moment that reveals the secret to weight loss, followed by a claim that weight loss is effortless on this special plan, and last ended with a diet plan that involves cutting calories and encouraging exercise.

MYTH: Severely restricting calories will lead to a longer life.

REALITY: Researchers found that by severely cutting calories, life could be prolonged in rodents and chimps. They don't know if the same results could be true for humans, but there are people who have dedicated themselves to a lifestyle of caloric restriction in exchange for a 130-year lifespan. In the few human studies, people were asked to cut their calorie intake by 25% of their usual intake for several years. Though their blood pressure and blood sugar levels improved, most could not maintain the severely limited diet. We think you are better off maintaining a healthy weight to reduce disease risk now, instead of chasing the elusive goal of living to be 130.

MYTH: Gimmicks, such as weight-loss soap, can speed weight loss.

REALITY: Gimmicks of any sort help lighten your wallet, not your body. In the example of weight-loss soap, which promises to penetrate the skin and remove body fat, if a weight-loss scheme sounds too good to be true, it is! Did you know a corset is being touted as an "external stomach bypass without the surgery"? Its manufacturer boasts that a cinched-in corset makes you feel uncomfortable if you eat a large volume of food. These are just two examples of the hundreds of wacky weight-loss gimmicks.

MYTH: Dietary supplements (like carbohydrate or fat blockers, over-the-counter stimulants, herbs, or minerals) speed weight loss.

REALITY: There is usually a theoretical basis for every supplement that claims to help you lose weight, but the theory usually falls short when put to the test. In one scientific review of weight-loss supplements, researchers concluded that most supplements lack a strong research base to produce long-term, sustainable weight loss. Plus, some weight-loss supplements contain stimulants that may elevate blood pressure or heart rate, which can be dangerous for many people. And most supplements come with a package insert that encourages following a calorie-cutting weight-loss diet along with the supplement.

MYTH: Menopause makes maintaining a healthy weight impossible.

REALITY: Hormonal changes at menopause can affect body composition—typically, there is an increase in fat storage in the abdomen—but by being vigilant about calorie intake and exercise, a healthy weight can be maintained. You may never have the body you had when you were 25, but you can achieve and maintain a healthy weight at any age.

Commonly Asked Questions About Weight Management

Is exercise more important than cutting calories for weight loss?

The simple answer is both are important, but for weight loss, decreasing calories is critical. Most of us can't out-exercise a high-calorie intake. Cutting calories is more important for weight loss, but exercise helps speed fat loss and is better for maintaining weight loss. So for weight maintenance, exercise seems to be the key. Ninety percent of the participants in the National Weight Control Registry reported exercising at least an hour every day to maintain their weight loss. Exercise has many benefits in addition to weight maintenance, and it behooves all of us to find time each day to be active.

To reduce calories, are snacks like veggie chips a healthy alternative to potato chips?

While veggie chips sound healthy, they can have more calories, fat, and sodium than other chips. Don't let the name of a product or the marketing on the front of the package lead you to believe a food is healthy. Read the Nutrition Facts label and focus on these two things: the number of servings in the package and the number of calories per serving. Then, think about the size of your typical portion and how this translates in calories. If you eat an entire bag of chips (veggie or otherwise) and the bag contains two or three servings per bag, you are getting many more calories than what is contained in a single serving. Being mindful of servings and the number of calories per serving can help you keep better control over the size of your portions.

Is green tea extract a good weight-loss supplement?

Hundreds of supplements with green tea extract claim to deliver dramatic weight loss. Don't believe it. While green tea extract is a mild stimulant that has the potential to increase metabolic rate, there is no evidence that the supplements will result in meaningful weight loss. Green tea extract could also increase the risk for liver damage. Enjoy drinking green tea, but be cautious with the supplements.

Having the Confidence to Maintain a Healthy Weight

Maintaining a healthy body weight means adopting healthy habits. With so many food choices, it can be overwhelming to change old habits, but if we keep doing what we've always done, we will get the same results. Scientific studies have proven that carrying excess weight has health risks, but carrying excess weight can also affect your quality of life. Being overweight or obese can make it harder to walk, for instance, and walking is one of the best exercises to maintain health and independence. Many of us love to travel, so being able to walk through airports, get on and off trains, and enjoy walking around our travel destinations will be hampered if we pack on extra pounds. If you can change only two dietary habits to maintain a healthy weight, they should be to right-sizing our meal portions and decreasing the frequency of snacking. Let's take a look at both in more detail.

Right-Size Your Portions

We are fortunate to live in a country where most of us have enough to eat, but the downside is that it's easy to eat too much. In addition, we waste a lot of food. Experts estimate that Americans waste almost 40% of the food supply every year. To keep portions in check, consider adopting a few of the following strategies, whether at home or dining out.

- Learn to recognize sensible portions. Dig out the measuring cups and pour a cup of cereal or 5 ounces of wine into your usual bowl or wine glass so you have a visual reminder of what a portion size looks like in your dishes. The sizes of our glasses and dishes also affect portion sizes. Behavioral research has shown that we drink more from short, wider glasses than from tall skinny ones, and we eat more from large dinner plates than smaller plates. We are not suggesting that you throw away your dishes and glassware and replace them with new stuff; just be aware of how visual cues can lead us eat or drink more than we need.

- Plan a weekly menu and shop accordingly. You don't have to be rigid and stick to the menu every day, but having a weekly menu and foods on hand to prepare meals can help cut down on the need to run to the store or a drive-through window, where impulse buying or oversize portions are more likely. Start by taking stock of what is on hand; look at your pantry staples and refrigerator and freezer contents and use what is already on hand as the basis for meals. A half a bag of frozen peas, a can of bean sprouts, leftover chicken, and day-old rice make for an easy fried rice dish that doesn't require you to purchase any new ingredients.
- Put your food on a plate instead of serving it family style, and leave food that's not plated on the counter or on the stove. More food on the table usually means more food consumed. If you are hungry after you've eaten, drink a glass of water and wait a few minutes for your stomach to communicate with your brain before going for seconds.
- Cook a big batch of your favorite foods and freeze it in individual containers to keep control over portions.
- When dining out, be mindful of the all-you-can-eat buffet. For many people, this type of buffet translates to "get your money's worth!" When faced with a buffet, take stock of everything on the buffet before loading your plate. Choose what you really want to eat and avoid the temptation to try everything. Instead of eating bacon, sausage, and ham from the breakfast buffet, choose one meat and move on. Buffets also trick us with variety. Research has shown that when faced with a greater variety of the same food, we eat more. For example, if there are five different pasta shapes, we eat more than if there is just one shape, even though they all taste the same.

- Don't be afraid to choose an appetizer as your entrée. Add a soup or salad, and you will have more than enough food to satisfy you.
- When half portions are an option, go for it. Some half portions are still enough to feed two people, but calories are kept in check—and you'll spend less money.
- If you drink, know what consitutes a serving of an alcoholic drink. Moderation is defined as one drink a day for women and two for men. A drink is a 5-ounce glass of wine, 12 ounces of regular beer, or 1½ ounces of 80-proof distilled spirits, like vodka, gin, or rum (see the figure below). What makes each of these a "drink" is that they all deliver the same amount of alcohol. The calories might be vastly different, depending on whether mixers are used with spirits, but the alcohol content is the same. Moderation reduces your risk of alcohol-related health and social problems. Alcohol consumption also tends to loosen your resolve to eat healthy by breaking down inhibitions making you more likely to reach for the wings and chips instead of the fruit and veggies when you are drinking.

WHAT'S A DRINK?

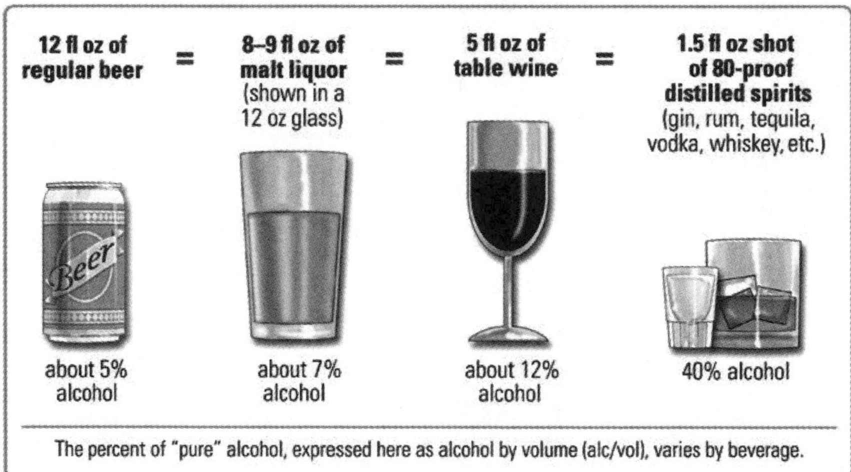

Source: What Is A Standard Drink?; National Institute on Alcohol Abuse and Alcoholism

Decrease Snacking

How many times do you snack during the day? When registered dietitian nutritionists tell people to eat multiple, mini meals throughout the day to curb hunger, many people forget the mini part and continue to eat three regular meals with added snacks. In Chapter 6, we talk about consuming protein throughout the day to support muscle building and maintenance. However, many people overconsume post-exercise snacks and sabotage the calorie-burning workouts. Snacking has become ubiquitous; many of us don't leave the house without an energy bar tucked in our purse or pocket. Instead of loading up on snacks, eat regularly spaced meals. When active, limit snacks to small portions to support your work out, not sabotage it.

Everyday Tips to Keep You on Track

Losing, gaining, or maintaining your weight require awareness and commitment. Weight creep happens, especially during winter months, when there's fewer opportunities for physical activity, so being vigilant is paramount. We've presented eating plans in Chapter 2 and exercise strategies in Chapters 5, 6, and 7, and here are some additional tips that can help you throughout the years.

- Monitor your weight. Make it a habit to weigh yourself several times a week, first thing in the morning. A study from the Duke Obesity Prevention Program found that weighing yourself every day leads to a greater adoption of behaviors that help control weight and greater weight loss compared with less-frequent weigh-is. But don't obsess over the numbers on the scale; it is normal for weight to fluctuate by a couple of pounds every day. The goal is to pursue a downward trend or to maintain your weight. For many older women who have been chronic dieters their entire lives, we say aim for good health, maintain your current weight, and learn to accept your body type and shape.
- Consider journaling. Among overweight, postmenopausal women, greater weight loss was achieved by those who kept a

food journal. Write down what you eat or use an app on your phone to log your food intake. This helps make you more mindful of food choices and portions, which is known to support weight loss. See the Useful Resources section on page 227 for more on digital tracking.

- Beware of athleisure wear. Sweatpants and yoga pants are for workouts and yoga occasions, but they don't give you much feedback if you are putting on pounds. Wear pants or jeans with a belted waist (no elastic) and use them to monitor your size. This is especially important around the holidays; if you have a pair of "Thanksgiving pants" (pants that you trot out each Thanksgiving because they are so big that you don't care how much you eat), ditch them!
- Don't deny yourself any food. Denial or deprivation makes you want it more. But remember that the second half of the cheesecake tastes just like the first half. So enjoy a few bites, but don't be a member of the clean-plate club, especially when it comes to desserts.
- Use fruits and vegetables to pump up the volume of your meals. When you add volume to meals, you will feel more satisfied, which can help to reduce calories from other foods. For example, add fruit to your cereal, include a side salad with an entrée, and put more veggies in every dish you make to increase its appetite-suppressing volume.
- Learn new cooking strategies. For example, try chopping mushrooms and mixing them with ground beef or turkey for a juicy, healthier burger, meatloaf, or taco filling. Mushrooms are rich in an amino acid that imparts umami, or the "fifth taste" (in addition to the tastes of sweet, sour, salty, and bitter).
- Set health goals, not weight goals. We've said this before, but focusing on your health is truly the most important goal. Weight loss often follows when health goals are reached.

Conversation With an Expert

James Hill, PhD, is an internationally recognized obesity expert and professor of pediatrics and medicine at the University of Colorado. His diet and fitness advice mirrors the content of this chapter. When it comes to diet, Jim describes his habits as "middle of the road. There are not things I totally exclude from my diet, and my philosophy is to eat reasonably healthy most of the time. I love good food, and we eat out frequently." He freely admits that "one of the smartest things I did was to marry a dietitian."

Jim stays active because he has seen "bad things happen to your body when you quit moving. I am 65 years old, and I see the consequence in my peers who are not physically active. It is not pretty. I also feel better when I am active." Jim aims for daily activity but admits he doesn't always succeed, especially when traveling. He also works on:

> just moving more during the day. Counting steps is a great way to track lifestyle activity. I work in a building with a fitness center, so the barrier to exercise for me is low. I live in a neighborhood where it is easy to walk to places rather than drive, and I try to get walking in every day. I live in a house with five levels, and I want to continue to be able to climb those stairs as I age. Being active—walking and cycling and being able to climb stairs—is important to me.

Through his research on obesity and weight loss and maintenance (the National Weight Control Registry discussed in this chapter is one facet of Jim's research), he translates his research by adopting "a small changes approach to nutrition and exercise to make a big difference in health and happiness. There are so many little things you can do and develop as habits to improve your lifestyle." Jim's book, *State of Slim,* was written to help people achieve and sustain a lifestyle that optimizes health and well-being—and produce weight loss.

Jim works with chefs to alter recipes and menus for improved public health but also for his own personal satisfaction. "Because I love to eat out so much, I am committed to helping restaurants be able to provide healthier alternatives. I have seen so many talented chefs who can make small changes to the foods they offer to make them healthier without losing the wonderful taste."

Jim reminds us that food and exercise go hand-in-hand. "To be able to really enjoy food, you have to do the exercise," he says.

How the Authors Manage Their Weight

Chris: I was a chronic dieter in high school. My mother encouraged me to drink grapefruit juice before meals, thinking the acidic fruit juice would burn the calories in the food eaten at the next meal and lead to weight loss. The only thing it did was make me dislike grapefruit juice. I maintain a BMI under 25 and have for 40 years; I monitor my weight daily, eat for good nutrition and enjoyment, exercise most days of the week, and am comfortable with my body type, which I describe as "good Eastern-European stockiness"!

Bob: I think I might just be too vain to allow myself to even get a little pudgy, so weight control has never been a problem for me. My biggest challenge is to keep winter weight gain to a minimum, and I usually manage that by finding ways to ramp up daily activity. Unlike during the summer and fall months, when I can work in the yard, I spend too many winter hours in front of my office computer. Eating less has never seemed like an enjoyable option for weight control, so I opt for moving more. In the winter, that means more time working out on the stationary bike or treadmill and with exercise videos, along with swim workouts at least 3 days each week. I find that if I can get in at least 7 hours of exercise each week, that's enough to minimize winter weight gain.

Useful Resources

Websites

BMI Calculator (www.nhlbi.nih.gov/health/educational/lose_wt/BMI/bmicalc.htm)
▷ *Online tool to calculate your body mass index by entering your height and weight*

Conscienhealth (http://conscienhealth.org)
▷ *A blog post that discusses obesity issues, from research to treatment in a respectful and sensitive manner*

Harvard T.C. Chen School of Public Health (www.hsph.harvard.edu/obesity-prevention-source/waist-circumference-guidelines-for-different-ethnic-groups)
▷ *Abdominal measurement guidelines for different ethnic groups*

Intuitive Eating (www.intuitiveeating.org)
▷ *Website, books, and podcasts by registered dietitian nutritionists Evelyn Tribole and Elyse Resch, that focuses on creating a health relationship among food, the mind, and the body*

National Institutes of Health (www.nhlbi.nih.gov/health/educational/lose_wt/index.htm)
▷ *Tools and resources to help you assess your weight and aim for a healthier weight*

National Weight Control Registry (www.nwcr.ws)
▷ *Research findings and tips from those who have successfully maintained weight loss*

Obesity Action Coalition (www.obesityaction.org/wp-content/uploads/prescription_medications.pdf)
▷ *Fact sheet on prescription medications and weight gain*

Books and Articles:

Bits & Bytes: A Guide to Digitally Tracking Your Food, Fitness, and Health by Meagan Moyer, MPH, RDN. Chicago: Eatright Press; 2017.
▷ *A guide to getting started with digital tracking of food and fitness habits*

"The Pima Paradox" by Malcolm Gladwell. *The New Yorker Magazine*. February 2, 1998. (http://gladwell.com/the-pima-paradox)
▷ *Enlightening article about the fight against obesity, with a look at several popular diet approaches*

State of Slim: Fix Your Metabolism and Drop 20 Pounds in 8 Weeks on the Colorado Diet by James Hill and Holly R. Wyatt. New York: Rodale Books; 2013. (www.stateofslim.com)
▷ *A 2-phase weight loss program for weight loss and maintenance, based on researcher's knowledge of what keeps Coloradans slim and fit*

CHAPTER

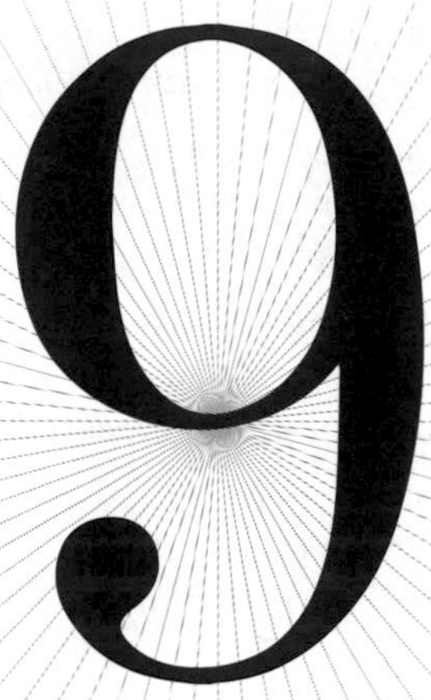

WHY SLEEP, STRESS, AND SOCIAL CONNECTIONS MATTER FOR OPTIMAL AGING

The Bottom Line

Getting sufficient sleep, managing stress, and developing and maintaining social connections are crucial to both our physical and mental health as we age. Here are some key points to keep in mind:

- **Sleep, both quality and quantity, can change as we age, but older adults still need 7 or 8 hours of sleep each night.**
- **For those who have trouble sleeping, developing a night-time routine to get ready for sleep and eliminating noise and light from the bedroom can help. This includes weekends too; avoid the urge to sleep in, and stick to your usual routine.**
- **For many adults, caffeine intake late in the day negatively impacts sleep quality, so avoid it if needed.**
- **Stress cannot be avoided, but it can be managed.**

- **Exercise is good for the body, for the mind, and for stress relief.**
- **Social connections are important for health and happiness as we age.**
- **Group activities, religious organizations, and community functions can all be sources of social support.**

ASSESS YOURSELF: IN REVIEW

Take the Assess Yourself quiz on the next page, and then read on.

If you are getting 7 or 8 hours of sleep each night, congratulations. That is the recommended amount of sleep for older adults. If the quality and quantity of your sleep has changed, you are not alone. Many older adults complain of sleep disturbances, and we will explain why that occurs and what you can do to get a more restful night's sleep.

Assessing the sources of stressors in your life is the first step to managing it. While stress can't be avoided at any age, many lifestyle choices can alleviate the negative effects of stress.

Social support is important at any age; loneliness is bad for your mental and physical health. For those of us who live far from family, activities such as volunteering or engagement with a religious institution can help fill the need for social connections.

Sam is a retired store owner. For 40 years, he owned and operated a furniture store, but he sold the business when he retired. He and his wife raised two daughters, and both have moved far away from home. His wife has an active life of community and church service and has encouraged Sam to become an active volunteer, too. Sam says he wants some downtime after 40 years of work and living on a schedule. When he had the store, he woke up at 6:30 every morning and was in the store by 8 AM, even though the store did not open until 10 AM. Closing time was 7 PM, and he usually got home about 8:30 PM. Now, in retirement, Sam stays up late watching movies and catching up on television shows that his daughters have recommend. He usually snacks when watching television: popcorn, chips, pretzels, nuts, and a beer or two. Although he

Assess Yourself: Sleep, Stress, and Social Connections

Have your sleep habits changed since you were 25?

☐ Yes
☐ No
☐ About the same

Is the quality of your sleep different, the same, or better since you were 25?

☐ Different
☐ Better
☐ About the same

Do you watch television in your bedroom before going to sleep?

☐ Yes
☐ No

Do you keep your tablet, ereader, or phone by your bed when you sleep?

☐ Yes
☐ No

Do you fall asleep quickly or does it take more than 20 minutes to fall asleep?

☐ Yes, I fall asleep quickly.
☐ It takes me a while to fall asleep.

What gives you stress in your life?

☐ Family dynamics
☐ Work-related stress
☐ Health stress
☐ Financial stress
☐ Other

Are you a caretaker?

☐ Yes
☐ No

If yes, for whom and how many hours a day do you estimate you spend on care-taking duties?

____

If you are a caretaker, do you view it as stressful?

☐ Yes
☐ No
☐ Sometimes

Do you have more, less, or about the same level of stress in your life compared with when you were 25?

☐ More
☐ Less
☐ About the same

How often do you interact with family (parents, siblings, children, etc)?

☐ Daily
☐ Several times a week
☐ Several times a month
☐ Several times a year

Do you wish you had more or less interaction with your family?

☐ More
☐ Less

Are you estranged from any family members?

☐ Yes
☐ No

If yes, is the estrangement a source of stress?

____

How many close friends do you have? Do you think you have just the right amount of friends, or do you wish you had less or more friends?

☐ The right amount
☐ I wish I had more
☐ I wish I had less

Are you actively engaged in life through work, hobbies, volunteer activities, and/or religious or spiritual activities?

☐ Yes
☐ No

Are you retired?

☐ Yes
☐ Yes, but I changed careers and work full time in another line of work
☐ Retired but still work part time
☐ No

often falls asleep in front of the television, he doesn't go to bed before 1 AM and then has restless sleep. He still wakes at 6:30 AM, although he tries to stay in bed until 8 AM. Sam complains that his sleep habits are off and that he feels tired all the time, even though he is not working. Sam has altered his normal routine, and it is taking a toll on him.

Introduction

Up to now, we've focused on food and physical activity to support good health. However, other factors can also have a big impact on optimal aging. In the late 1980s, two social scientists, John Rowe and Robert Kahn, developed a model of what they termed "successful aging." To age successfully, one needed to reduce risk of disease and disability; ensure high levels of physical and cognitive function;and remain an active participant in life. Feelings of joy, happiness, optimism, and energy, as well as life satisfaction are tied to optimal aging. What can older adults do to capture those feelings? How well you sleep, how you deal with stress, and being socially connected can all contribute to overall wellness—which includes your food and fitness—and, ultimately, to successful aging.

Clarifying the Science on Sleep, Stress, and Social Connections

Is there enough sound evidence to say that getting adequate sleep, controlling stress, and having strong social ties can positively affect aging? The answer is yes, to all three. Following is an overview of the science and what is known about each factor.

Sleep

Remember when you were a kid and your parents had to force you to go to bed? Something changed in adulthood, and most of us now look forward to going to sleep! There is good reason for wanting to sleep. Sleep is restorative; it helps the nerve cells in your brain repair and reconnect. It also helps keep the immune system strong. In addition, researchers have linked sufficient sleep to better blood sugar control, better heart health, happier moods, and lower body weight. Leptin, a hormone that helps us feel full, drops when we don't get enough sleep. This can leave us feeling hungry, leading to greater food intake and weight gain if not countered with physical activity.

Sam's story illustrates how a change in his daily routine is changing not only his sleep schedule, but also his eating and activity. All of these factors will influence his health if he doesn't make some changes, starting with his sleep. You'll hear more about Sam later in this chapter.

Adults need 7 or 8 hours of sleep a night, but many older adults complain that they don't sleep as well as they did when they were younger. It is hard to say if changes in sleep are a direct result of getting older or if they're caused by diseases, medicines, or lifestyle choices. As with most things in life, it is probably a bit of everything. As we age, sleep time shortens and sleep patterns become more disturbed; as we grow older, we spend more time awake during the night and have a harder time falling back to sleep. It is unclear why this happens, but two proposed theories involve declining hormone levels and changes to our normal 24-hour rhythms. Declining levels of testosterone in men and estrogen in women may influence sleep. As they transition through menopause, 40% to 60% of women complain of trouble falling asleep and experience more fragmented sleep. Hot flashes and night sweats also contribute to poor quality and quantity of sleep among older women.

The circadian rhythm also changes. This normal 24-hour cycle of wake/sleep gets disrupted with aging and makes our normal timing feel off. Anyone who has traveled across time zones has experienced jet lag, which is another way of saying your normal body clock or circadian rhythm is out of whack. Two tiny, pinhead-sized regions in the brain near the optic nerve process daylight and start the 24-hour cycle each morning. When that gets disturbed, our sleep patterns can also be disturbed. So it's true that normal aging may contribute to sleep problems, but there are many other things that can affect a good night's sleep.

Obesity, heart problems, asthma, allergies, gastrointestinal problems, urinary issues, chronic pain, depression, and anxiety can affect sleep, as can some of the medications used to treat these conditions. Specifically, selective serotonin reuptake inhibitors, bronchodilators, and nondrowsy allergy medications can make it harder to get quality sleep. Then there are the lifestyle choices: caffeine, nicotine, and alcohol consupmtion can negatively affect sleep in some older adults.

Caffeine, the most widely consumed drug in the world, is known for its ability to keep us sharp, focused, and awake. A moderate amount of caffeine is defined as about 400 milligrams a day (roughly the amount in three to four small cups of brewed coffee), according to the American Medical Association's Council on Scientific Affairs, but even at a moderate dose, caffeine has the ability to alter sleep quality.

In the United States, 85% of the population consumes at least one caffeinated drink a day, and older adults may respond differently to caffeine than younger adults when it comes to sleep. Caffeine before sleep may increase the time it takes to fall asleep and decrease total sleep time. More women than men report sleep problems when using caffeine. Many aging adults have noticed that they used to be able to drink coffee late in the day with no effect on sleep, but as they've gotten older, even small amounts of caffeine in the late afternoon keep them tossing and turning. Not everyone has trouble sleeping when consuming caffeine, however, and by now, you should know how caffeine affects you. You probably do your best to avoid it if you are a caffeine-sensitive person. Caffeine is sneaky in that it is found in some foods, beverages, and over-the-counter medicines that may surprise you. Medicines for migraine or tension headache relief often contain caffeine—as much as or more than a cup of premium coffee. The amount of caffeine in a food or drink is not required to be listed on the Nutrition Facts label; remember, caffeine is a drug, not a nutrient. Everyone knows that caffeine is in coffee and coffee drinks, but caffeine is also showing up in everything from waffles (wired waffles) to beef jerky (perky jerky). Adjectives such as invigorating, energized, or spark might be hints that the product contains caffeine. The box on page 234 lists some caffeine-containing foods that might surprise you. For more information on how much caffeine is in your favorite beverages or foods, see the Useful Resources section on page 246.

Popular Foods that Contain Caffeine

Decaffeinated coffee (some decaf coffees have trace amounts of caffeine, while some have up to 20 milligrams)

Tea (hot, iced, fresh brewed, instant, or bottled)

Chocolate milk

Hot chocolate

Chocolate candy

Some regular and diet soft drinks, including cola, lemon-lime, root beer, orange, and cream sodas

Coffee-flavored ice cream

Energy waters

Caffeinated gum and mints

Some snack foods, from potato chips to sunflower seeds to popcorn; some snack-food makers add caffeine to foods

Stress

Janet works full-time as a continuing education coordinator at a university. When she was 55, Janet's parents relocated to be near her. Janet is divorced and has three sons, two of whom live at home. One son dropped out of college and has a minimum-wage job, and the other son is a senior in college. Her parents are in their early 80s, and both have chronic health problems and expect Janet to take them to doctor's appointments, help them shop for groceries, and manage their medications. One of Janet's sons has a child with his girlfriend; the couple did not marry and are no longer together, but they share custody of Janet's granddaughter, so Janet also has childcare responsibilities. Janet feels her life as a caretaker is overwhelming. She is not just of the sandwich generation (caring for elderly parents and her own children), she is a club sandwich, caring for parents, children, and grandchild. Janet has let her own health slide; she no longer goes to the university fitness center, and most meals are grab-and-go from the school vending machines or drive-through fast food on her way home from her parents' apartment.

Stress is a scary word. Everyone experiences stress, so let's set the record straight—stress cannot be totally removed from our lives, but it is possible to learn ways to manage and cope with stress in a positive, healthy way. Stress isn't all bad; some stress can help motivate us to try new things and conquer our fears. This type of stress is called eustress, as opposed to bad stress or distress. Even the most seasoned public speaker or elite athlete experiences stress before taking the podium or entering a sports competition. How stress is handled is what counts. Janet's story might sound familiar. Many of us put the needs of others ahead of our own, and while that is sometimes necessary, it can be a major source of stress that negatively impacts health.

Stress takes many forms, from physical trauma at one extreme to daily hassles at the other. When humans perceive a life-threatening stressful event (eg, a car swerving into your lane, severe turbulence on an airplane, or an unexpected loud noise), the fight-or-flight response kicks in: our brains signal an immediate response to increase breathing, heart rate, and blood pressure and to sharpen vision and hearing to get the body ready to respond appropriately. Everyone has felt the surge of adrenaline and cascade of physical changes that occur during acute stress. After the initial response, a secondary phase kicks in; the brain signals the adrenal glands, two tiny organs that sit on top of the kidneys, to secrete another stress hormone called cortisol. These two systems help prepare us to deal with a life-threatening challenge. When the threat has passed, the brain reacts with the rest-and-digest phase as the body returns to normal. This reaction to stress was

Health Effects of Chronic Stress

- Altered immune function
- Weight gain (high circulating levels of cortisol make you hungry)
- Increased blood sugar
- Gastrointestinal problems
- Insomnia
- Anxiety
- Depression
- Muscle tension, especially in the neck and shoulders
- Headaches
- Impaired cognitive function, including memory

first described by Walter Cannon, a physiologist, in 1915. Cannon's work was expanded on in the 1950s by Hans Selye, who coined the term *general adaptation syndrome*. In addition to the fight-or-flight stage described by Cannon (Selye called this the alarm stage) and the return to homeostasis, Selye proposed that the body can become exhausted if the stress is chronic. In other words, if cortisol continues to circulate in the bloodstream in higher than normal levels, adverse effects can occur. The potential health problems associated with chronic stress are listed in the box on page 235.

The America Psychological Association (APA) conducts an annual survey called "Stress in America". According to the most current report, these are the top five stressors:

- money,
- work,
- family responsibilities,
- personal health concerns, and
- health problems affecting the family.

Many of our modern-day stresses are chronic. These may include worries about financial security during retirement, safety concerns in an uncertain world, caregiving responsibilities for elderly parents or young grandchildren, personal health problems, and grief over the loss of loved ones; all of these examples of ongoing stress can take a toll on our health. While these stressors can't be changed, coping strategies can be used to help alleviate their negative effects.

Psychologists suggest that coping strategies to deal with stress can run the gamut from less to more adaptive. Less adaptive strategies include anger, denial, blaming others, alcohol or drug abuse, and overeating. About 40% of people in the APA survey reported overeating unhealthy foods in response to stress during the 1 month peroid before the survey. Adaptive strategies include humor, problem solving, religious coping, social support, and altruism. A great example of altruism as a coping strategy is the nonprofit organization Mothers Against Drunk Driving (referred to as MADD). The organization, which educates and protects against drunk driving, was founded by a mother whose daughter was tragically killed by a drunk driver to help her cope with her loss and subsequent stress.

With aging, resilience might just be the most important personal characteristic that can be developed for optimal aging. The ability to reduce stress by being adaptable in the face of adversity can go a long way toward coping with the stresses that will come our way as we age.

Social Support

Esther is a 75-year-old widow who lives in her own home but is considering moving to an apartment in a retirement community in the southwestern United States. For 53 years, she lived with her husband in the Midwest and raised four children there. She has nine grandchildren and sees them frequently, but after a lifetime of living in a cold climate, she wants a change. She has reconnected with some old college friends who live in Arizona, and after a week-long visit with them, she talked to her children about moving to the same retirement village. During her visit, she learned that there might be part-time employment teaching knitting and needlework, two of her lifelong passions. Her children don't want her to sell the family home and are discouraging her from making a major life change at her age. Esther is in good health but feels her life revolves around taking care of her grandchildren. She wants time to explore a new phase of her life. Before her husband's death, she had never lived alone, and she has spent her life taking care of others. She has few friends where she lives and feels isolated, and she wants more social engagement with others her own age.

Social support takes many forms; family, friends, involvement in religious institutions, civic and personal clubs (eg, formal organizations, like Kiwanis and Rotary, or informal groups, like book clubs or bridge groups), and volunteerism are all types of support that offer social connections. Having social connections contributes to good health by decreasing the risk of high blood pressure, heart disease, diabetes, depression, and dementia. Social support is so crucial to health that social isolation and loneliness increase mortality. Esther has a need for social connection. Although she loves her interactions with her children and grandchildren, she longs for more interaction with people closer to her own age and wants to pursue her own interests and hobbies. With technology, such as cell phones and social media sites, Esther can stay connected to her family when separated by long distances. Still, family makes up the front line of support for aging adults, so it is understandable that Esther's children are concerned about her moving to a new environment hundreds of miles away.

It's important to know that those who live alone can be healthy; living alone and being lonely are two different things. Loneliness has been described as a public health problem, and one in three older adults report being lonely. Loneliness and social isolation change physical health by increasing inflammation and decreasing production of the antibodies that fight infections. In contrast, social support networks and physical activities are significantly associated with self-rated good health, even into very old age. In other words, people who have social support rate their health as better compared to those who have few social interactions. Social support can also act as a buffer to stress.

The most revealing fact about social support and how it affects optimal aging comes from the Harvard Study of Adult Development, which began in the 1930s by tracking Harvard undergraduate students and young men in Boston, and he has continued for more than 75 years. Robert Waldinger, MD, the current director of the study, says older adults might be surprised at the study's findings. For example, participants didn't derive happiness from health or wealth; instead, it was the relationships they developed during their lives that gave them joy. The men who were more socially connected to family, friends, and community were healthier and happier, and they lived longer. A link to Waldinger's blog and TED talk on social support is found in the Useful Resources section on page 246.

What about social connections through technology? The Pew Research Center reports that six out of every ten adults over the age of

65 go online, and about half have high-speed connections. Those in the younger age group of 65 to 69 years have even higher usage rates, similar to that of the general population. A little over three-fourths (77%) of older adults have cell phones, but fewer have smartphones. While smartphones aren't as commonly used in this age group, tablets and ebook readers are. Both are popular with older adults, similar to the rates of use among younger individuals. About half of those over 65 years of age use social networking sites, and those who do use them say they connect with the people they care about almost every day.

Still, there are some challenges to using new technologies for social connectivity. Physical challenges, such as poor vision and diminished manual dexterity, can make reading small screens or manipulating keyboards more difficult. Some older adults remain skeptical about the benefits of technology, but those who dive in and use technology find it becomes an integral part of their life. Last, learning new technologies can be hard. Some of us, like Bob, are early adopters who embrace the newest smartphone, computer programs, or apps, and others, like Chris, use technology daily but get anxious when it is time to replace a smartphone or update to a new program. For those of us in the latter category, it helps to have social support to show us how to use the new technologies.

Confronting Myths About Sleep, Stress, and Social Connections

MYTH: We need less/more sleep as we age.

REALITY: We need about 7 or 8 hours of sleep each night, the same amount as we did when we were younger.

MYTH: There is nothing older adults can do to improve their sleep habits as they age.

REALITY: Older adults can do many things to improve sleep, including sticking to a regular schedule for going to bed and waking up in the morning. Other strategies for improving sleep are covered later in this chapter.

MYTH: All stress is associated with negative health outcomes.

REALITY: It's normal to feel stress over many of life's situations, and occasional stress isn't harmful to your health. However, when stress is chronic, there doesn't seem to be end in sight, and you haven't developed coping strategies, stress can have physical and mental consequences.

MYTH: Men need fewer interactions with friends and family than women do.

REALITY: According to Robert Waldinger, MD, director of the Harvard Study of Adult Development, which has tracked the lives of more than 700 men for more than 75 years:

> Year after year, we asked about their work, their home lives, and their health—trying to determine what makes for a meaningful and healthy life. From this study, one important lesson about what makes for the good life emerges time and time again. Simply put, good relationships keep us happy and healthy.

Commonly Asked Questions About Sleep, Stress, and Social Connections

Are sleep medications safe for all older people?

Both prescription and over-the-counter sleep aids might be effective in the short term. Talk to your doctor about your concerns regarding sleep. If he or she recommends a sleep aid, always take it as directed and use the lowest dose possible. Always tell your doctor about other medications you are taking to be sure there are no drug or dietary supplement (such as melatonin) interactions. If you use a sleep aid and need to get up during the night to use the bathroom, sit up slowly and sit at the edge of the bed for a few seconds before getting out of bed. The drug might make you unsteady and cause a fall, leading to an injury or worse.

Can leisure-time activities contribute to physical activity recommendations?

Absolutely. It just depends on what you count as leisure-time activities. As many as 36% of adults engage in no leisure-time physical activity, so think about adding small bursts of active time to your usual fitness routine. For example, gardening, walking the dog, watching your favorite television show while pedaling an exercise bike or walking on a treadmill, or simply keeping exercise bands or weights near your favorite reading chair and doing a few exercises every 15 minutes can all add up.

My mind is always racing, and while I would like to meditate or practice yoga, I'm not sure I can.

The key word is in the question—practice! Yoga and meditation are both practices, and like anything else that is new or different, it takes patience and practice. Try an app for meditation; there are many free apps (such as Headspace) that guide you through a 10-minute meditation session. It isn't easy at first, but with practice, it gets easier. It is the same with yoga; give it a try.

Having the Confidence to Manage Sleep, Reduce Stress, and Strengthen Social Connections

Strategies for Improving Sleep

The best habit older adults can follow for good sleep is a regular sleep/wake cycle. We introduced Sam, a retired store owner, earlier in this chapter. Sam has altered his normal routine by staying up until the wee hours of the morning and forcing himself to stay in bed past the time his body tells him to wake up. We aren't suggesting that Sam keep the exact same hours as he did when he was working, but by honoring his body's normal rhythm and getting on a schedule, Sam is likely to get better-quality sleep and still have time to do all of things he enjoys. Sam might try shifting his bedtime and wake-up times by half an hour instead of dramatically altering his normal rhythm.

Other tried-and-true strategies include the following:

- Keep your bedroom dark, cool, and quiet. Try room-darkening shades, and hide the LED lights from the television, ereader, tablet, phone, alarm clock, or other sources. If you have your phone next to your bed, either put it on silent or keep it in a drawer in a bedside table so you aren't disturbed by light, beeps, or alarms coming from it throughout the night. To keep your bedroom cool, consider using a ceiling fan, even in the winter months. If you can't turn off the noises outside your bedroom (barking dogs, traffic noises), consider a white-noise machine or a steady sound, like a fan blowing, to muffle outside noise.
- Avoid caffeine and nicotine and limit alcohol consumption before going to sleep. Alcohol might seem like a relaxant, but drinking can cause restless sleep.
- Relax before sleep. Try reading a book, listening to music, or taking a warm bath.
- Regular exercise enhances sleep quality, but heavy exercise in the hours before bed does not. Move your hardest workout to earlier in the day.
- Avoid heavy meals or snacks before sleep, especially if you have acid-reflux disease. High-fat foods, gas-forming foods, chocolate, coffee, and alcohol can cause worsen reflux.

Strategies for Managing Stress

Remember, you are never going to live a stress-free life, but there are many options for dealing with stress. The annual APA survey found the most common stress-relieving activities to be:

- exercise, such as walking
- listening to music
- surfing the internet
- watching television or movies
- reading
- spending time with family

Other activities that help us deal with stress include practicing relaxation techniques, such as massage or meditation; engaging in hobbies; and volunteering.

While these may be the most common activities reported to be helpful in dealing with stress, we think exercise is the best remedy. We've talked a lot about the physical benefits of exercise in previous chapters, but the mental side of exercise is just as important for optimal aging. Physical activity has been shown to reduce anxiety and depression; improve mood and self-esteem; improve sleep; and, of course, help alleviate stress. Just one exercise session can make us feel calmer and less anxious. Active people are 45% less likely to develop symptoms of depression than those who are sedentary. Regular exercise has been found to be just as effective—or perhaps more so—than antianxiety drugs for many people. Exercise can also lower cortisol levels, which are elevated with chronic stress. Exercise scientists have studied the relationship between physical activity and the psychological constructs of control, self-efficacy, and competence. Exercise not only improves physical health but also helps us gain confidence in setting and achieving goals.

Strategies for Strengthening Social Connections

With aging, many adults no longer have social connections through work, but there are many things you can do to develop and build social engagement:

- If you have a partner, enlist his or her help. If your partner or spouse is socially engaged, you will be more likely to develop social connections.
- Be a joiner. If you love to read, find a book club. If your hobby is flying model airplanes, there is probably a club with like-minded individuals. Church or community groups are always looking for volunteers. Start small, and take on a task you enjoy.
- Look to your community for free concerts, art shows, or craft fairs, and attend the events to meet new people.
- Go out and play. Find a golf group, an exercise class, or a walking partner to get active and be social.

- Use technology to stay connected with friends and family; Facetime with your nieces, nephews, or grandchildren if you don't see them in person very often, and friend them on social media sites. Learn to text; email is old school to your grandchildren!

Conversation With an Expert

Nancy P. Kropf, PhD, is professor and dean of the Byrdine F. Lewis School of Nursing and Health Professions at Georgia State University in Atlanta. Her degrees are in social work, and she knows from professional and personal experience that a healthy diet and physical activity are great antidotes to the challenges of aging. She explains, "The research on exercise, even in moderate amounts, is very persuasive. There is no disputing the evidence that exercise helps physically, mentally, and emotionally as we age." Nancy has been a runner since she was 19, so that gives her a 38-year history of being active. She says:

> I am very drawn to stories about active older adults, such Grandma Gatewood, who had 11 children and 23 grandchildren and was the first woman to hike the entire Appalachian Trail at the age of 76, and Olga Kotelko, a 97-year-old track-and-field star who holds 37 world records (the last one earned at the age of 95). Although not everyone will be super performers like these two women, their stories inspire me and give us examples of what is possible in later life.

Nancy is a pescatarian (one who eats fish but no meat) and enjoys following the research on the health benefits of plant-based diets. She says, "I did not come from a family that practiced great nutrition habits, and I have tried to inform myself about healthier food habits that support my physical activity and put me on a path to optimal aging." Nancy sticks to three meals a day and usually has a smoothie for lunch. With her busy life as dean of a college that trains health professionals, she sets a good example for colleagues and students.

Goal-setting is an important part of Nancy's quest to stay healthy as she ages. She says, "I had a midlife goal of running a marathon before I turned 50—which I did 6 weeks before my 50th birthday. Now, at 56, I've run 20 marathons in 19 different states." She loves outdoor activities and hikes and trail runs at her getaway home in the mountains of north Georgia.

Nancy knows the path to good health as we age is never straight; there are bumps in the road, and detours are possible. But, she adds, "there are so many benefits to eating well and staying active. Yes—it's often hard to find time to grocery shop, cook, and work out...but there are lots of ways to make better decisions about our health—even if we can't commit to training for a marathon." Those healthy habits can make us sleep better, act as an outlet for stress, and keep us socially connected, all of which are important for optimal aging.

How the Authors Manage Sleep, Reduce Stress, and Strengthen Social Connections

Chris: I get 7 or 8 hours of sleep each night and wake only when the dogs bark. Living in the country cuts out street noise and city lights, which helps me get quality sleep. I find exercise to be the best mood elevator and stress reliever ever discovered. When I worked as a dietitian in cardiac rehab, the cardiologist encouraged the staff to walk or jog with the patients. That was my introduction to exercise, and I haven't stopped being active since 1977. I also find that 10 minutes of meditation each day helps me to be mindful of life's blessings. I have a supportive spouse, siblings, and many nieces and nephews for social support, and I also have a large network of friends. I am an active volunteer in my profession and community, and activities continue to expand my social connectivity.

Bob: I love to sleep and have learned from experience that caffeine and alcohol disrupt my slumber. I have also learned that while sleep aids can be helpful on a periodic basis, taking them on successive nights is a recipe for poor sleep quality and developed a reliance on the sleep aids. I have also learned to distinguish good stress from bad stress. As with most people, I spent most of my life not differentiating between the two, and lumping all types of stress together as one big negative. Once I became aware that some kinds of stress are healthy—the stress of exercise is a good example—I was able to reduce my overall stress level. After all, the stress of trying to accomplish something new and challenging can be a good stress, compared to the stresses of relationship issues or money woes. Like many other men, I don't feel the need for constant social interaction or support and rely on my wife to keep me engaged with friends and family more often than I might on my own.

Useful Resources

American Psychological Association (www.apa.org/news/press/releases/stress/index.aspx) and (www.apa.org/helpcenter/stress-body.aspx)
▹ *Summary of the Stress in America survey and the effects of stress*

Center for Science in the Public Interest (https://cspinet.org/eating-healthy/ingredients-of-concern/caffeine-chart)
▹ *Caffeine content of common foods and beverages*

Exercise Is Medicine Initiative (www.exerciseismedicine.org/support_page.php/older-adults)
▹ *Description of some benefits and resources for exercise for older adults*

Harvard Health Publications (www.health.harvard.edu/staying-healthy/understanding-the-stress-responsewww.health.harvard.edu/staying-healthy/understanding-the-stress-response)
▹ *Information about the stress response and techniques for handling stress*

National Institute of Mental Health (www.nimh.nih.gov/health/publications/stress/index.shtml)
▹ *Fact sheet on the five things you should know about stress*

National Institute of Neurological Disorders and Stroke (www.ninds.nih.gov/Disorders/Patient-Caregiver-Education/Understanding-Sleep)
▹ *Discussion on the importance of sleep and suggestions for improving sleep*

National Sleep Foundation (https://sleepfoundation.org)
▹ *Tips on getting a good night's sleep*

MacArthur Foundation (www.macfound.org/tags/aging)
▹ *Insightful articles on many aspects of aging, including social connections*

What Does the Good Life Actually Look Like? (http://robertwaldinger.com/about)
▹ *Lessons from the longest-running (75 years) study on happiness*

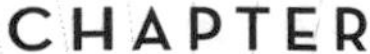

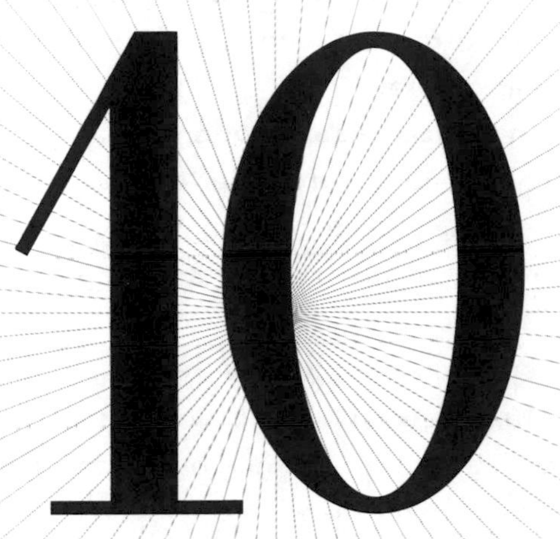

FOOD AND FITNESS STRATEGIES FOR ILLNESS AND INJURY

The Bottom Line

Although many people bemoan getting older and the challenges that it brings, we like to think of aging as a privilege that not everyone gets to experience. While your chronological age can't be changed, your risk for chronic diseases that are often associated with aging can be greatly reduced via food and fitness strategies tailored to your individual circumstances. Following are some key points to keep in mind:

- **The most common chronic conditions that are associated with aging are also the most preventable.**
- **It is never too late for older adults to improve their diets, increase their physical activity levels, or engage in preventive measures, like vaccines and regular screenings, to stay healthy at any age.**
- **Be an active partner with your health care provider. If you experience a health problem or sustain an injury, take the time to**

learn about the condition and ask questions about how food and fitness can help you manage your condition.

- **Not every health problem is preventable, but you can control how you react to disease, illness, and injury and come back even stronger than before.**
- **Prescription medications are modern miracles, but they shouldn't replace healthy eating and regular physical activity.**
- **There are no magic foods or miracle exercises, but healthy eating patterns and regular activity can help halt the progression of some diseases.**
- **Some dietary supplements show promise for supporting blood sugar level management and blood vessel, heart, bone, joint, and brain health, but they should be used with diet and exercise, not as a substitute for them.**
- **In this chapter, we share our own personal stories of health challenges that deterred but did not stop us from striving to return to good health and resume our fitness goals.**

At 54, Chris was diagnosed with breast cancer. After the shock of a cancer diagnosis wore off and the surgery and treatments were over, she faced 5 years of drug therapy that came with its own side effects (elevated cholesterol, bone density loss). Chris had no family history of cancer. She was fit and ate well, so the diagnosis was a big emotional blow. After the treatment, Chris resumed running despite an arthritic hip that was always annoyingly sore after a long run. The running felt like good healing therapy, despite the discomfort. She tried glucosamine-chondroitin and over-the-counter nonsteroidal anti-inflammatory drugs (NSAIDs), but the pain worsened. When the pain became so severe that even walking produced a limp, she sought advice from an orthopedist. The doctor said that an MRI (magnetic resonance image) showed severe arthritis and joint degeneration. She prescribed NSAIDs, physical therapy, and a cortisone shot, which worked for a little while, but the pain came back and the limp got worse. Chris tried acupuncture for 8 weeks—anything to prevent a total hip replacement. Everything seemed to help for a little while, but eventually the hip joint was damaged to the point where surgery was the best alternative. At 62, she had a total hip replacement. The surgery was successful, but her surgeon advised to avoid high-impact exercise, like running, mixed martial arts, and ski jumping. (She would miss running, but the other two activities were never going to happen!) Having a hip replacement meant changing her usual exercise routine. While she had previously enjoyed running, walking and cycling became the new normal aerobic exercise. She found recreational cycling to be so much fun that she planned a bike and barge trip to Europe and cycled from Amsterdam to Bruges. This demonstrates that despite disease, injuries, and aging, new routines can turn out to be exciting adventures.

At age 30, Bob was diagnosed with atrial fibrillation (Afib), the most common type of electrical disturbance of the heart muscle. Millions of Americans, mostly over age 60, suffer from Afib, and most are able to manage the problem with blood thinners, such as Coumadin (warfarin). The biggest risk with Afib is a stroke caused by small blood clots that can develop in the heart because it does not empty efficiently. Normally, the two smaller upper chambers of the heart (the atria) contract in unison, pushing blood into the two larger chambers that lie below (the ventricles). When the ventricles contract, their contents are sent to the lungs for oxygenation—the job of the right ventricle—and to the rest of the body—the job of the left ventricle. The atria normally contract in unison because a group of pacemaker nerve cells in the atria send out an impulse about once every second (making for a normal resting heart rate of roughly 60 beats per minute). In Afib, other cells also send out impulses, so instead of contracting rhythmically, the atria contract irregularly, disrupting the normal function and capacity of the heart. When he was younger, Bob's Afib was just an occasional nuisance, but after he turned 40, the episodes of Afib became more frequent. By the time he turned 50, his Afib was persistent, and Bob struggled with symptoms of lightheadedness, shortness of breath, and overall fatigue. Bob's cardiologist prescribed a number of different medications, none of which helped. Over the next few years, Bob underwent three cardiac ablations, a procedure in which doctors pass long catheters into the heart through the femoral vein in the legs and then create scar tissue to stop the extra impulses from causing the atria to contract. Those efforts gave Bob only temporary relief; the Afib returned a few months after each procedure. At age 57, Bob decided to undergo an open-heart operation known as the MAZE procedure to surgically create lines of scar tissue that restore normal control of atrial contraction. For a physically active guy like Bob, recovery from open-heart surgery was a frustrating process that proceeded at an agonizingly slow pace. Bob faithfully stuck to his recovery plan, starting 2 weeks after surgery with a 5-minute treadmill walk at 0.5 mph—truly a snail's pace. Six months later, Bob was back to his normal exercise routine, and now, almost 10 years later, he remains free of Afib.

Introduction

Even with the best eating habits and a smart exercise plan, stuff happens. Active adults sometimes need joint replacements, break bones, or struggle with life-altering diseases, such as cancer or heart disease. In addition, accidents happen that have nothing to do with our food or fitness; however, being in good health can help shorten and improve recovery, when injury strikes. Chris believes her quick recovery from hip replacement was a result of being fit before surgery. Bob's adherence to a schedule of regular physical activity and a healthy, varied diet were not new behaviors, so after open-heart surgery, his return to business as usual occurred naturally. Many people, especially older adults, struggle after major surgeries to cope with the rigors of recovery while trying to embrace new dietary and physical activity habits. Without the necessary internal motivation and external guidance, many fail to modify the lifestyles that may have contributed to a need for surgery.

Good nutrition and fitness can certainly reduce the risk of chronic disease, but even active adults can develop high blood pressure, diabetes, or heart disease. These health challenges might slow us down, but they do not have to deter us from our food and fitness goals. For many, a health scare is what it takes to overhaul eating habits or start a serious fitness program. Medicine has a name for this: *secondary prevention,* a process for developing strategies to slow down the progress of the disease or injury with the goal of getting back to good health. For example, monitoring high blood pressure and treating it with a combination of diet, exercise, and medication can greatly reduce the risk of subsequent stroke. For those who have undergone cardiac bypass surgery, lifestyle modifications (as part of a cardiac rehabilitation program) can help keep the heart strong and reduce the risk of a heart attack or repeat heart procedures. This chapter will discuss secondary prevention strategies to keep you well after a health problem has been identified.

We often have a tendency to blame ourselves for things we might have done to cause cancer or heart disease, but the bottom line is that bad health outcomes can happen to anyone. It can be tempting to blame it all on bad genes. As the saying goes, "Choose your parents carefully." However, genetics isn't destiny, and everyone can improve their diet and exercise habits to soften the effects of family history of disease. We also want to point out that the most common chronic diseases (heart disease, stroke, high blood pressure, obesity, and some cancers) are also the most preventable diseases, and all respond positively to healthy eating and physical activity.

ASSESS YOURSELF: IN REVIEW

Take the Assess Yourself quiz on the next page before reading on.

Let's start with the questions on smoking. The good news is that cigarette smoking rates are low among older adults, but 10% of men and 8% of women over the age of 65 do smoke. Quitting is hard, but people can and do quit smoking. You are never too old to quit, and the health benefits from quitting are significant at any age. Cigars are not a safer alternative to cigarettes because they contain the same cancer-causing compounds as cigarettes. Many options are available to help smokers quit; if you are a smoker, have a serious talk with your doctor about strategies to help you quit for good.

Assess Yourself: Lifestyle

Do you smoke cigarettes?

☐ Yes

☐ No

If no, were you a former smoker?

☐ Do you smoke cigars?

☐ Yes

☐ No

If yes, how often?

____

Do you have any chronic health conditions?

☐ Yes

☐ No

Do you get an annual flu shot?

☐ Yes

☐ No

If you are over the age of 65, have you had a pneumonia vaccine?

☐ Yes

☐ No

If you are over the age of 60, have you had a shingles vaccine?

☐ Yes

☐ No

Have you had a colonoscopy to screen for colorectal cancer?

☐ Yes

☐ No

If you have had a colonoscopy, have you followed your doctor's advice for repeat screening?

☐ Yes

☐ No

For women, have you had regular mammograms to screen for breast cancer?

☐ Yes

☐ No

If you drink alcohol, do you do so in moderation?

☐ Yes

☐ No

Moderate alcohol intake is defined as one drink per day for women and two drinks for men (see Chapter 8 for what is meant by "one drink"). The fact is that it is easy to over-pour a drink, and many imported or craft beers contain more than 5% alcohol, meaning that one beer might have the equivalent alcohol of 1½ drinks. While many of us enjoy drinking alcohol in social settings, we don't recommend that you start drinking if you don't drink already. Although some health benefits may be associated with alcohol consumption, you can do other things for good health besides drinking.

We're going to cover food and fitness for chronic diseases in the next section, but it is important to discuss prevention with vaccines and cancer screenings as part of the self-assessment review. We encourage you to talk to your doctor about getting an annual flu shot.

About 70% of older adults get a flu shot each year, and we hope you are among that group. We've heard some people say (and we bet you have, too) that the flu shot gave them the flu. That can't happen; it may be that someone was exposed to the flu and got sick before the vaccine had time to afford protection. It takes about 1 to 2 weeks for a flu shot to ramp up immunity. There is also a chance that you might have been exposed to a different strain of the flu virus than the one you were vaccinated against. Those are not good reasons to avoid getting a flu shot, especially for older adults with chronic diseases.

The Centers for Disease Control and Prevention (CDC) recommend that those over 60 years old get a shingles vaccine to prevent shingles and shingles-related nerve pain (called postherpetic neuralgia). The CDC also recommended that those 65 years and older get vaccinated against pneumonia. It only takes one or two shots in our lifetime to protect against pneumonia. The latest numbers show that only 61% of those over 65 have gotten the pneumonia vaccine, so put that on your list of things to talk to your doctor about at your next visit.

Two cancer screenings are recommended for adults over 50: for all, a colonoscopy for colorectal cancer, and for women, mammography to screen for breast cancer. Only about 52% of men and women in the 50- to 64-year age group have had a colonoscopy, though the percentage is higher, about 70%, aomng older age groups. Screening for colorectal and breast cancers can be lifesaving; Chris is glad she had regular annual mammograms, as a routine screening caught her early stage cancer, which was treatable and has a high cure rate.

Clarifying the Science on Aging and Chronic Disease

Chronic diseases tend to occur more frequently among older adults; indeed, age is a major risk factor for many diseases. About 80% of older adults have at least one chronic condition. The most common diseases are high blood pressure, cardiovascular disease, diabetes, osteoporosis, osteoarthritis, and cancer. Obesity is also classified as a chronic disease and is covered in detail in Chapter 8. While cognitive decline is not a disease, we also will cover some strategies to keep your aging brain healthy. For each health concern, we'll include a brief description of the condition, suggested foods or dietary plans for its management, supplements that show promise to augment dietary strategies, and activity suggestions to complete the routine. To be clear, the information presented is not meant to replace your doctor's instructions or to suggest that you should ditch your prescription drugs. This information is presented only to enhance your knowledge of how you can be an active partner in your health care and not simply be the recipient of medical advice.

Prehypertension and Hypertension

A healthy or normal blood pressure is 120/80 millimeeters of mercury (mm Hg). The top number is the systolic pressure or the force of the heart contraction as it pumps blood out of the heart to the body. The bottom number is the diastolic pressure (if you can't remember which number is which, think of the letter "d" for the "down" number of the 120/80), which is the pressure inside the heart and major arteries between heart beats. Both numbers are important, so all adults should know their usual blood pressure. However, don't panic if you use the free blood pressure cuff at the drug store; if you've been running errands and plop down in the chair to take your blood pressure, it is likely to be a high with a single reading. Blood pressure fluctuates throughout the day to meet the demands of activity; systolic pressure normally rises during physical activity. So, it is not unusual to have a high blood pressure reading the first time it is taken. In addition, a phenomenon called white-coat hypertension results in a high blood pressure reading when it is first taken in a doctor's office.

If you have been diagnosed with high blood pressure, it is likely that your doctor prescribed a medication but said little about how diet and exercise could complement your treatment. High blood pressure has been described as the most prevalent yet the most modifiable disease in older adults. Some doctors have even called it a neglected disease. The key to managing high blood pressure is working with your health care provider to understand how to monitor and manage your blood pressure to avoid serious consequences, such as heart attack, heart failure, stroke, peripheral artery disease, and kidney disease. People who manage their high blood pressure increase their life expectancy by 5 years over those who don't. Food and fitness can have a major impact on managing blood pressure, even if you take medications.

Dietary Advice

The healthiest eating plan for treating high blood pressure is the Dietary Approaches to Stop Hypertension (DASH) eating plan. Research shows that adopting a DASH eating plan lowers blood pressure in men and women of all ages and races. As we discussed in Chapter 2, the plan is rich in fruits, vegetables, whole grains, and low-fat dairy. The plan calls for choosing lower-sodium foods but also encourages foods rich in the minerals potassium, calcium, and magnesium; that is where the fruits, vegetables, and low-fat dairy foods come in. They are natural sources of the minerals that can help lower blood pressure and at the same time are low to moderate in sodium content. Sodium is part of salt (sodium and chloride), and most health organizations, including those that emphasize blood pressure lowering, suggest limiting salt to 6 grams a day (1 teaspoon, which translates to 2,300 milligrams of sodium) for all adults and children ages 14 years and older. Adults with prehypertension and hypertension are advised to further reduce sodium to 1,500 milligrams per day for even greater blood pressure reduction. Reducing salt doesn't mean going salt free—sodium is a needed nutrient. A glass of milk has about 120 milligrams of sodium, which sounds like a big number, but consider that a burger and fries from a quick-service restaurant contains about 1,100 milligrams of sodium, almost half of our entire daily need for the mineral. Not everyone is salt sensitive, meaning that a high sodium intake results in an increase in blood pressure. However, we do know that people over 50 and those diagnosed with high blood pressure are more likely to be salt sensitive. It is estimated that 90% of Americans consume higher-than-recommended intakes of sodium, so it is a good idea to assess your intake and try to come close to the recommendations for good health. About 75% of our sodium comes from packaged and restaurant foods, not from the salt shaker.

While there is no one best food to lower blood pressure, the table below shows some foods that supply minerals that can help to lower blood pressure, and the box on the next page provides smart strategies to reduce sodium intake.

FOODS TO HELP LOWER BLOOD PRESSURE

Calcium Sources	Potassium Sources	Magnesium Sources
Milk (dairy, soy, almond, cashew, rice)	Tomato and tomato products (sauce, paste, soup)	Cooked spinach
Yogurt (regular, Greek, and Icelandic)	Bananas	Beans (black, kidney, white, navy, lima)
Cheese	White and sweet potatoes	Pumpkin seeds
Cooked leafy green vegetables	Milk	Nuts (almonds, Brazil nuts, cashews)
Canned salmon and sardines	Lentils	Peanuts and peanut butter
Cottage cheese	Cooked spinach	Avocado
Tofu	Beans	Edamame
Calcium-fortified orange juice	Peas	Soy milk
	Dried fruit	Wheat bran cereals
	Broccoli	Whole wheat bread
	Citrus fruits	Brown rice
	Kiwi fruit	
	Cantaloupe	
	Dried plums (prunes)	
	Beef, poultry, fish	
	Soy and veggie burgers	
	Nuts	

Source: Office of Dietary Supplements, National Institutes of Health

Supplements that Show Promise

Dietary supplements that may be helpful in managing high blood pressure include coenzyme Q10 and hibiscus tea. Check Appendix B on page 291 to learn more about these and other popular dietary supplements: what they are, why they are used, effectiveness, and other things to consider if you use the supplement.

Strategies to Reduce Sodium Intake

Not all high-sodium foods taste salty; cheese, especially processed American cheese and cheese spreads, can be high in sodium.

Drain and rinse canned beans to reduce their sodium content by about 40%.

Limit use of condiments, such as ketchup, soy sauce, and Worcestershire sauce.

Be aware that added sauces and seasonings can add a lot of sodium to foods like frozen vegetables.

Read labels and compare sodium between products. On the Nutrition Facts label, next to the sodium number is the percentage of the daily value. If that number is 20% or higher, it is a high-sodium food; if it is 5% or less, it is a low-sodium food.

Eat fewer salty meats, such as cured meats (pepperoni, salami, cold cuts, sausage, and bacon).

Cook at home with fresh ingredients or no-added-salt frozen foods as often as you can to reduce sodium; season with herbs and spices instead of salt or salt-containing blends.

Don't be fooled by seasoning blends that sound salt free: blends such as lemon pepper, nature's seasoning, Italian seasoning, and many others list salt as the first ingredient.

Choose unsalted nuts for snacks or when cooking.

Make your own salad dressing with good quality olive oil, balsamic vinegar, and garlic; it is practically sodium free.

Check labels for chicken and turkey and choose those that have no added salt water or saline broth.

Reduce portion sizes to also reduce sodium content.

Physical Activity to Help Manage Hypertension

About 20% or one in five people with hypertension do not receive any advice on exercise from their health care provider, despite evidence that regular exercise is a powerful way to reduce blood pressure.

Cardiovascular Disease

Cardiovascular disease (CVD) is a broad term encompassing diseases of the heart and blood vessels. While there are many types of CVD, two that disproportionately affect older adults are coronary artery disease and stroke. Heart disease is the number one cause of death for men and women in the United States. Heart disease is a broad term for several heart-related conditions, but we will focus on coronary heart disease, also called coronary artery disease, as that affects many over 50.

The heart is a muscle, and like all muscles, it needs a blood supply to provide oxygen and nutrients. After all, the heart is a muscle that never stops working. Tiny blood vessels called coronary arteries (some as small as the lead in a pencil) feed the heart. If these small arteries become too clogged with fatty deposits, the stage is set for angina (chest pain) and heart attack, as shown in the illustration of coronary artery disease.

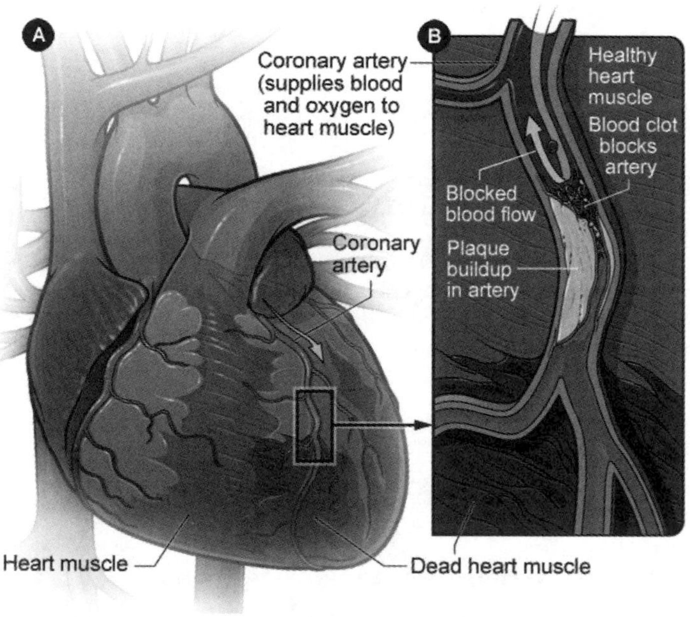

Source: National Institutes of Health, National Heart, Lung, and Blood Institute.

Coronary artery bypass surgery, angioplasty, or stent placements are procedures that allow blocked arteries to be bypassed (hence the name "bypass surgery") or to be held open with tiny implants called stents. These procedures have been lifesaving; in 2000, there were 519,000 bypass operations in the United States. Having a coronary procedure is, however, not the end of the story. Healthy dietary patterns help keep the arteries from getting reblocked, and exercise strengthens the heart muscle to reduce the need for repeat surgery in the years ahead.

Some risk factors for CVD can't be changed: increasing age, gender (men have more coronary heart disease than women), and heredity. However, heredity isn't destiny; being overweight or having diabetes ups the risk and interacts with inherited genes for heart disease. The risk factors you can control include smoking, high blood cholesterol, high blood pressure, overweight and obesity, type 2 diabetes, and physical activity.

Stroke is another type of CVD. Of the two types of stroke, ischemic stroke is the most common. Ischemia means lack of blood flow to body tissues, usually from blocked arteries, so an ischemic stroke is like a heart attack in the brain. The other type of stroke is hemorrhagic stroke, which is caused by a burst blood vessel in the brain, most often as a result of uncontrolled high blood pressure.

Dietary Advice

Any of the four healthy eating plans discussed in Chapter 2 are good for reducing heart disease risk. The Mediterranean diet gets high marks from researchers as the most well-studied plan to reduce heart disease. A study conducted in Spain called PREDIMED, found that following a Mediterranean diet was associated with fewer major cardiovascular events, such as heart attack, stroke, and death from heart disease. The main feature of the diet is that it is rich in unsaturated fats (extra virgin olive oil and nuts) and high in phytonutrients. Foods central to the plan include fish, olives and olive oil, fruits, vegetables, legumes, whole grains, and a little red wine. People who followed the Mediterranean eating plan had improved risk factors for heart disease, including improved blood pressure, blood lipid levels, inflammation and insulin sensitivity, and oxidative stress.

Foods to eat less of include those with *trans* fats and saturated fats. *Trans* fats, described in Chapter 2, have already been significantly reduced in the US food supply. You can find *trans* fats listed on Nutrition Facts labels. Because amounts below 0.5 gram per serving can be rounded to zero on the label, it's a good idea to check the ingredient list for partially hydrogenated oil, which is a clue that the food still contains some *trans* fat. The box on page 260 shows foods that may still contain *trans* fats.

Saturated fats are also discussed in Chapter 2, but the main culprits in raising heart disease risk appear to be the saturated fats found in fatty meats (highly marbled steaks, beef or pork ribs, ground chuck, and sausage) and tropical oils, such as palm kernel oil and coconut oil.

Foods that May Contain *Trans* Fat

Stick margarine
Butter
Refrigerated canned biscuits
Refrigerated canned cinnamon rolls
Refrigerated ready-to-bake cookies
Muffin mixes
Frozen pie crusts
Doughnuts
Pastries
Frozen pizza
Processed American cheese

Supplements that Show Promise

Flax seed oil, omega-3 fatty acids (fish oil), and fiber have all shown some benefit for heart health when combined with diet and exercise. Check Appendix B on page 291 to learn more about these and other popular dietary supplements: what they are, why they are used, effectiveness, and other things to consider if you use the supplement.

Physical Activity to Help Manage Coronary Heart Disease

Being physically active at moderate intensity levels for just 2 hours each week lowers the risk of coronary artery disease by a whopping 50%. For lighter physical activity, the risk reduction is 12% to 20%, which is still significant for those prone to heart disease.

It should be clear to you by now that among the many benefits of regular physical activity is a reduced risk of heart disease. Some of the reasons for that reduced risk are obvious: improved blood lipid profile, better control of blood pressure, enhanced blood sugar control, and lower body fat. In addition, as we become more fit, our heart muscles become stronger pumps, better able to withstand the stresses of heart disease. But if you do need surgery at some point, having a stronger heart is clearly better, and it is also important to help you to recover quickly and completely. For those who have suffered a heart attack or who have had bypass surgery or stent placement, research clearly shows that regular physical activity in the form of cardiac rehabilitation improves overall quality of life, reduces future hospital admissions, and lowers mortality (death) rates.

Prediabetes and Type 2 Diabetes

Almost one quarter of Americans age 65 and older have diabetes. Of the many forms of diabetes, the most common is type 2 diabetes. Type 1 diabetes, most often diagnosed in children, adolescents, and young adults, requires a lifetime of insulin replacement. We will focus on type 2, as that is the type that most often affects older adults. Almost everyone who has type 2 diabetes had prediabetes, that is, blood sugar levels that are higher than normal but have not reached the threshold for a diabetes diagnosis. With a smart eating and exercise plan, prediabetes can be reversed and may never advance to diabetes. The two most common tests for diagnosing diabetes are fasting blood sugar ("fasting" means you can have no food or drink for at least 8 hours before the test) and glycated hemoglobin A1c (HbA1c) (which requires no fasting). The HbA1c test is an estimate of average blood sugar levels for the past 2 or 3 months. The table below shows common blood tests and results used to diagnose diabetes.

DIAGNOSING DIABETES

Diagnostic Test	Normal	Prediabetes	Diabetes
Fasting blood sugar	Less than 100 milligrams per deciliter	Between 100 and 125 milligrams per deciliter	Greater than 125 milligrams per deciliter
Hemoglobin A1c	Less than 5.7%	Between 5.7% and 6.4%	6.5% or above

Source: Diagnosis of Diabetes and Learning About Prediabetes, American Diabetes Association, www.diabetes.org/are-you-at-risk/prediabetes/

In most cases, prediabetes and early-stage type 2 diabetes are symptom free, but the damage from uncontrolled high blood sugar can be life threatening. Asymptomatic individuals with a body mass index > 25 and one or more risk factors for diabetes, such as family history, should be tested routinely. People with diabetes are twice as likely to have a heart attack than those without diabetes. Diabetes, if not controlled, can damage the eyes, kidneys, skin, nerves, and blood vessels. The good news is that treating diabetes by controlling blood sugar, blood lipids, and blood pressure levels, and keeping the levels as close to normal as possible may prevent or delay complications. Doctors work with a team of professionals, including registered dietitian nutritionists (RDNs) to offer diabetes self-management education, which helps individuals manage their diabetes.

Dietary Advice

There is no such thing as a "diabetic diet." As we have learned more about the disease and tools for its management have increased and improved, people with diabetes no longer have to follow a rigid meal plan. A healthy eating pattern, like the ones we recommend in Chapter 2, works for diabetes management. People with diabetes need to eat regular meals with all types of carbohydrate distributed between meals and snacks, but self-monitoring has eliminated the need for restrictive plans. An RDN who is also a certified diabetes educator (CDE) can help customize a meal plan that will promote blood sugar control and prevent complications.

Some fiber-containing foods should be a part of everyone's meal plan, especially those with diabetes. Foods that contain a special kind of dietary fiber called soluble fiber, such as pulses or legumes (beans and peas) and oats, help lower blood sugar and stabilize blood sugar and insulin levels. Legumes are also higher in protein than other vegetables, and they increase satiety to help with weight management. Legumes (also known as pulses) are so nutritious and valuable as a food worldwide that 2016 was named the International Year of Pulses by the Food and Agriculture Organization of the United Nations. Foods that are rich in soluble fiber are shown in the box on the next page.

Sugary drinks, such as sugar-sweetened soft drinks, fruit drinks, fruit punch, sweetened tea, and energy drinks, supply calories from

Foods Rich in Soluble Fiber

Apples
Barley
Beans (black, kidney, navy, great northern, and other starchy beans)
Blueberries
Flax seeds
Lentils
Nuts
Oatmeal
Peas (chickpeas, black-eyed peas, and other starchy peas)
Prunes

added sugars with little or no nutrients, and they tend to be quickly absorbed into the bloodstream in a way that elevates blood sugar levels more rapidly than sugary foods. Although sugar is not off limits to people with diabetes, it's important to be mindful of proper portion sizes and consider the nutrient quality of any beverage or food with added sugars. On the other hand, there is no need to buy special foods, such as diabetic candies or cookies. One of the most important things you can do if you have elevated blood sugar levels is control your weight—losing just 7% of body weight (that would be 14 pounds for someone who weighs 200 pounds) has a significant impact on lowering blood sugar and controlling diabetes.

Supplements that Show Promise

Alpha-lipoic acid and fiber supplements are two supplements that show promise in helping to manage blood sugar levels and possibly reduce complications of diabetes. Check Appendix B on page 291 to learn more about these and other popular dietary supplements: what they are, why they are used, effectiveness, and other things to consider if you use the supplement.

Physical Activity to Help Manage Diabetes

Physical activity is associated with lower blood sugar and HbA1c levels, as well as improved insulin sensitivity. When our muscles are active, glucose from the blood (blood sugar) enters muscle cells more rapidly than when they are at rest, providing an energy source to sustain muscle contractions. For those who battle high blood sugar, regular physical activity is an essential part of controlling blood sugar levels. Along with a following proper diet and taking medications, engaging in moderate- to vigorous-intensity physical activity at least 3 days each week (avoid consecutive days of inactivity), and strength training 2 days a week is recommended for adults with type 2 diabetes.

Osteoporosis

"Osteo" means bone, and "osteoporosis" means porous bone. Among people with this condition, the desnity and strength of bone decreases to the point where a broken bone can occur more easily. While all bones can be affected, the wrist, hip, and spine are often the most likely to break. If you've gotten shorter with age, you might have lost bone in your spine, thus reducing your height. It is not an unusual response to say "I used to be..." when asked about your height. For example, if you are 1½ inches shorter than you were at the age of 20, you might be at risk for osteoporosis. One in two women and one in four men over the age of 50 years will break a bone due to osteoporosis. The risk is real, so we should all treat our bones with respect! While osteoporosis affects more women than men, it is not a woman's disease. Men have larger skeletons and don't lose bone as early in life as women, but by ages 65 to 70, men lose bone at a similar rate as women. As life expectancy has increased for men, so has the risk for developing this bone disease.

Just as prediabetes happens before diabetes is diagnosed; osteopenia or low bone density is the first step toward osteoporosis. Low bone density doesn't mean osteoporosis will occur, but it can serve as a warning to incorporate lifestyle changes to strengthen and protect your bones. Your doctor can order a bone-density test to determine your risk. The National Osteoporosis Foundation recommends that men and women have a bone-density test at age 65, but the test should occur earlier if you have risk factors for osteoporosis. Your doctor might do a risk assessment is his or her office, and you can be proactive by asking about your bone health at your next visit. It is also important to tell your doctor about any other medicines that you take, as several drugs can be harmful to bones. Aluminum-containing antacids and proton-pump inhibitors used to treat indigestion and gastric reflux can cause bone loss, and because these drugs can be bought without a prescription, you might not think to mention them to your doctor. Several prescription drugs are also hard on bones: aromatase inhibitors, used for cancer treatment, and corticosteroids, used to treat asthma and severe inflammatory conditions, are two examples. Both drugs are taken long term, so make sure to ask your doctor about what you can do to protect your bones if you take these drugs. The National Osteoporosis Foundation has a doctor's visit checklist that you can print out and take to your next visit to get the conversation started. A link to the form is found in the Useful Resources section on page 284.

Dietary Advice

In Chapter 4, we talk about bone-building nutrients and provide lists of foods rich in key bone-building nutrients. To recap, calcium– and vitamin D–rich foods fall into the bone-building category. Dairy foods, fish (such as salmon with soft bones), and some fruits and vegetables are good choices to help protect your bones. Fortified foods, such as orange juice or ready-to-eat breakfast cereals, can also increase your calcium intake. Emerging research points to bone benefits of olive oil, flax seed oil, soybeans, blueberries, and dried plums (prunes). Another easy and inexpensive way to boost calcium intake is nonfat dry milk powder; think of it as the original protein powder! Adding a tablespoon to smoothies, hot cereal, cream soups, mashed potatoes, or casserole dishes give you 50 milligrams of calcium, along with protein as an added bonus. Vitamin D is harder to get in foods, so unless you like fatty fish or cod liver oil, look for vitamin D–fortified food, such as ready-to-eat breakfast cereals, milk, yogurt, and orange juice. Mushrooms exposed to ultraviolet light can also be a source of vitamin D.

Supplements that Show Promise

Many of you may already take calcium and vitamin D supplements (more on taking calcium supplements is found in Chapter 4 and in Appendix B on page 291), but look more closely at your diet before you simply add more calcium or vitamin D. For example, a multivitamin mineral supplement for women over 50 usually contains about 200 milligrams of calcium and 1,000 International Units of vitamin D, so combined with foods, you might be hitting the target for both nutrients. If you find you cannot get enough calcium or vitamin D from your diet, take the lowest dose that will get you to the recommended intakes. Check Appendix B on page 291 to learn more about these and other popular dietary supplements: what they are, why they are used, effectiveness, and other things to consider if you use the supplement.

Physical Activity to Help Manage Bone Health

Both weight-bearing and muscle-strengthening exercises are especially good for bones. Regardless of your age, your bones will adapt to the stress put upon them by gradually becoming stronger. For example, walking, jogging, hiking, stair climbing, tennis, pickle ball, dancing, and other weight-bearing activities stress bones with each and every step. The same is true with strength training, which places a different kind of stress on bones but also results in stronger bones.

Osteoarthritis (OA)

Joint wear and tear is a common side effect of aging. One in five adults will be diagnosed with arthritis, and everyone over the age of 60 probably has some arthritis, even if it isn't bothersome. The joints most commonly affected by arthritis include the neck, spine, hips, knees, fingers, and thumbs. When two bones come together to form a joint, a substance called cartilage helps coat the ends of the bones to keep them from rubbing together. The entire joint is surrounded by a capsule, and the lining of the capsule produces a fluid that lubricates the joint, similar to the oil that the *Wizard of Oz*'s Tin Man used to keep his joints moving. Unfortunately, injecting our joints with oil to keep them moving and free of pain isn't an option!

As we age, our cartilage can break down, leading to joint inflammation or arthritis ("arthro" means joint, and "itis" means inflammation). There are several types of arthritis, but OA is the most common type. It can occur in younger people too; athletes who have repeated injuries to joints can develop arthritis at an early age. Keeping the joint healthy involves strengthening the muscles around it to keep it stable.

Dietary Advice

The best thing you can do to manage OA is maintain a healthy weight. First, excess weight puts a strain on the spine, knees, and hips. In one study, just a 1-pound weight loss was found to unload 4 pounds of stress on the knee joint among individuals with OA. Second, fat produces compounds called cytokines, which cause inflammation and further damage joints. Reducing body weight is considered the most effective modifiable risk factor for OA. We've given you a lot of reasons to maintain a healthy weight in Chapter 8, so let's add reducing pain from osteoarthritis to the list of benefits.

Cartilage contains collagen, a protein that supports body tissues. Vitamin C is important in making collagen, so getting adequate vitamin C every day can help produce this important protein. More isn't better, though; there is no evidence that extra vitamin C helps us make more or better collagen. Vitamin C–rich foods are discussed in Chapter 4.

A hallmark of OA is inflammation, so anti-inflammatory foods might be beneficial. The eating plans outlined in Chapter 2 feature anti-inflammatory foods. Specific foods that show promise in fighting inflammation are included in the box at right.

Foods that May Help Reduce Inflammation

Apples
Berries
Cherries
Coffee
Green leafy vegetables
Nuts
Olive oil
Oranges
Pomegranates
Salmon
Strawberries
Tomatoes
Tuna

Supplements that Show Promise

Glucosamine and chondroitin are the supplements that are top of mind for many with OA. Glucosamine is found in cartilage, and chondroitin is a carbohydrate that helps draw in and retain water in cartilage. The two are often taken together to ease OA pain. Researchers wanted to know if they worked to reduce pain in patients with knee OA, so they conducted what is known as the gold standard of research: a placebo-controlled, double-blind study. The Glucosamine Arthritis Intervention Trial (GAIT) found that long-term (24 months) use of a placebo, a prescription medication, and a combination of glucosamine-chondroitin all had similar outcomes; there were beneficial reductions in knee pain with each treatment, but they were not statistically significant. We think these results speak to the difficulty of evaluating the effectiveness of dietary supplements—arthritis is a fickle disease. Older adults with OA might feel fine one day and then experience pain the next. It is hard to pinpoint exactly what works to ease pain. Talk to your doctor if you want to try glucosamine and chondroitin, but if you don't have relief of symptoms after 3 months on the supplement, it probably isn't going to work for you. Increasing the dose won't help, and the supplement will not rebuild cartilage. Check Appendix B on page 291 to learn more about these and other popular dietary supplements: what they are, why they are used, effectiveness, and other things to consider if you use the supplement.

Physical Activity to Help Manage Osteoarthritis

It sounds counterintuitive to exercise when arthritis pain flares up, but the Arthritis Foundation advises regular activity to help ease pain, improve energy levels, and increase muscle. For example, strengthening leg muscles helps support the knee and hip joint and provide a stable, strong base. Range-of-motion exercises can improve joint flexibility; stretching, yoga, and tai chi are also useful to manage OA. Many older adults like water aerobics, which can take the stress off an aching joint and still provide an aerobic activity. The physical activity guidelines mentioned throughout this book are also relevant to those with OA. Moderate aerobic exercise—150 minutes each week (or 75 minutes of vigorous exercise)—along with two weekly sessions of strength training will help spark weight loss and strengthen muscles. Losing just 5% of body weight—that's 7 1/2 pounds for a 150-pound person—has been shown to reduce pain and improve function.

Cancer

There are about 15.5 million cancer survivors in the United States. Researchers are beginning to learn not only how improving diet and activity level can help people feel better as they transition from cancer patients to cancer survivors, but also how diet and exercise might help reduce cancer recurrence. While it isn't yet clear exactly which types of cancers benefit most from changes to food and fitness routines, both the American Institute for Cancer Research and the American Cancer Society recommend diet and exercise as part of a healthy lifestyle. The American Cancer Society has developed long-term guidelines to help doctors provide care for cancer survivors. Currently, guidelines are available for breast, prostate, head and neck, colon, and rectal cancers, and additional guidelines are in the works.

Dietary Advice

The same guidelines for cancer prevention are useful for cancer survivors. In general, the guidelines mirror the recommendations that we discussed in Chapter 2. These include:

- Choosing an eating plan that focuses on fruits, vegetables, whole grains, and legumes to provide vitamins, minerals, and fibers;
- Eating less red meat and trying to avoid processed meats;
- Limiting alcohol intake, knowing that heavy intake increases the risk for many cancers; and
- Keeping calories in check to maintain a healthy weight.

Here's an easy tip: Try to fill at least half of your plate with fruits and vegetables at every meal to get the phytonutrients tied to cancer prevention as well as key vitamins, minerals, and fiber. Fruits and vegetables also provide antioxidants.

Food safety is important for all of us, but depending on your treatment, your immunity may be lowered as you recover from cancer. To stay healthy, practice basic food-safety strategies: clean, separate, cook, and chill. Put those principles into action by doing the following:

- Wash hands thoroughly before and after food preparation.
- Keep hot foods hot and cold foods cold.
- Cook food to the right temperature; using a meat thermometer is preferable to eyeballing it. Using a thermometer also prevents overcooking.
- Remember the 2-hour rule; cooked foods and restaurant leftovers should not be allowed to be sit out at room temperature for more than 2 hours to prevent growth of bad bacteria. Refrigerate as soon as possible.
- Avoid raw milk, raw cheeses, and unpasteurized juices.
- Wash all fruits and vegetables before preparation, even if you are not eating the skins.
- Separate meat from produce in your grocery bags and refrigerator, and use separate cutting boards for meat and produce.
- Wash reusable shopping bags.

Dietary Supplements

Some friends and family members may suggest dietary supplements to prevent cancer recurrence. However, there is no evidence that any supplement can prevent (or treat) cancer, as much as we wish that were true. A multivitamin or mineral supplement may give you some peace of mind that you are filling nutrient gaps, but always check with your doctor before taking any supplement. Check Appendix B on page 291 to learn more about popular dietary supplements: what they are, why they are used, effectiveness, and other things to consider if you use the supplement.

Be aware that the effectiveness of cancer maintenance drugs can be affected by some dietary supplements.

Physical Activity for Cancer Survivors

Moderate exercise can improve fatigue, anxiety, and self-esteem for cancer patients. Exercise also has a secondary benefit for cancer survivors; it can help prevent heart disease, diabetes, and osteoporosis. Cancer survivors are more prone to these diseases than those who have never had cancer. In addition to all the health benefits of regular physical activity, research shows that among cancer survivors, recurrence is lower and longevity is extended in those who are physically active.

Depending on the type of treatment and how much time has elapsed after chemotherapy or radiation therapy, start slow with exercise. If you have anemia as a result of treatment, you may tire easily. Skin irritation from radiation may be aggravated by chlorinated water in swimming pools or hot tubs.

Cognitive Decline

"Where did I put my keys?" "What was the title of the movie I saw last week?" "I really like that actor, you know the one, what's her name?" These are questions adults ask themselves as they move into their 50s and beyond. How many of you have explained away your forgetfulness as a senior moment but secretly worried that you were developing a more serious memory impairment? Just as muscle changes with age, so does the brain. Beginning in the 40s, the brain starts to shrink. There are fewer nerve cells, and some of the connections in the brain can break. In addition to these normal brain changes, diminished blood flow to the brain means less oxygen to help with mental sharpness. The good news is that these are normal age changes, not signs of dementia or Alzheimer's disease. So don't panic when you can't remember what you ate for dinner last night or the name of the restaurant where you forgot what you ate!

We often use the computer analogy to explain our trouble, remembering things by saying our hard drive is full. The difference is that the brain still has plenty of storage capacity; we just have a harder time retrieving the information stored there.

Dietary Advice

In Chapter 2, we described the Mediterranean-DASH Intervention for Neurodegenerative Delay (MIND) diet as an emerging area of research for keeping the brain sharp. This eating plan, like the others we recommend, is rich in brain-healthy foods. Vegetables (especially green leafy vegetables), nuts, berries, beans, whole grains, fish, poultry, olive oil, and red wine are recommended in the plan. It also suggests limiting red meat, butter and stick margarine, cheese, pastries, sweets, fried foods, and fast foods. The research is not conclusive that this dietary pattern will prevent all cognitive decline, but a healthy diet may help. In addition to the foods recommended in the MIND eating plan, there are other nutrient-rich foods that older adults should include in their eating plans.

Lutein (pronounced loo-teen) is a nutrient present in green leafy vegetables, egg yolks, and avocados that appears to be tied to cognition. Lutein is a plant pigment, and along with another plant nutrient, zeaxanthin (pronounced zee-uh-zan-thin), it is deposited in the retina of the eye. Lutein and zeaxanthin are the only plant pigments found in high concentrations in the eye. Researchers have known for a while that lutein and zeaxanthin are important in slowing the development of age-related macular degeneration. However, researchers were surprised to find that older adults with higher levels of lutein in their retinas also had better cognition than those older adults with lower levels of lutein. Lutein is present in dark green (such as kale, spinach, broccoli, green peas), yellow (such as corn and summer squash), and orange (such as pumpkin and winter squash) vegetables. It is also found in egg yolks and avocados, and the fat found naturally in those foods help to increase lutein's absorption. Because egg yolks and avocados are rich in many of the nutrients in short supply in most older adults' diets, we suggest adding these foods to your healthy food list for cognitive function.

Dietary Supplements for Cognitive Function

If you've never heard the term *nootropics* (new-troh-picks), you've not seen the many advertisements for brain supplements that claim to increase alertness, reduce memory loss, and boost intelligence. The term is derived from the Greek word for acting on the mind, and these "smart drugs" are gaining a foothold with everyone from computer gamers to aging adults worried about memory loss. Most of the supplements are mixtures of various medicinal plant compounds and natural stimulants (eg, caffeine and herbal stimulants like green tea extract or ma huang). While many of these compounds have the promise to improve alertness, they are sold as dietary supplements, which means they are not subject to testing for efficacy before being sold. The advertising on websites and television are slick and convincing. Some supplements even provide clinical research to support their claims, but these examples are mostly animal research or findings taken out of context to promote a product. We suggest that you save your money and skip "revolutionary" products that claim to make you smarter.

One supplement that does have a more promising track record (ie, based on sound research) is citicoline. It was originally used in Japan as a treatment for strokes. Food is not a good source of citicoline or CDP choline; only a small amount is found in organ meats. Within the brain, citicoline has several functions. First, it helps stimulate the production of cell membranes. Second, citicoline increases the production of the neurotransmitters that have been shown to increase attention, focus, and memory. Research pertaining to memory loss is still scant, but it is promising. Check Appendix B on page 291 to learn more about this and other popular dietary supplements: what they are, why they are used, effectiveness, and other things to consider if you use the supplement.

Physical Activity for Cognitive Function

While the evidence for smart drugs may not be strong, it is clear that exercise (especially aerobic exercise) is beneficial. Regular physical activity can slow the rate of cognitive decline and even reduce the risk of developing more serious dementia.

Confronting Myths About Aging and Chronic Disease

MYTH: Exercise can't help me if I am diagnosed with a chronic disease.

REALITY: On the contrary, the American Medical Association and the American College of Sports Medicine launched the Exercise Is Medicine program to illustrate that physical activity not only helps prevent disease but should also be part of the prescribed therapy to treat disease. Exercise helps us not only physically but mentally. It is a great stress reliever and can make you feel less anxious about your health problems, so there is good reason to be active, even if you have a chronic disease.

MYTH: If I don't have any symptoms, I must be fine.

REALITY: We wish that statement was true, but many disorders, like heart disease, high blood pressure, and early stages of cancer, can be symptom free. In fact, high blood pressure is called the silent killer because it often goes undetected. If you truly want to be healthy as you age, screening and early intervention are key. It is easy to get your cholesterol levels or blood pressure checked at a health fair or walk-in clinic at a drug store, so don't put it off.

MYTH: I can't do anything to prevent injury as I age.

REALITY: Injuries can happen, but there some common-sense strategies to avoid injuries. Falls are the leading cause of injuries among older adults, and maintaining balance can go a long way to prevent injuries. Focus on the strategies in Chapter 7 related to flexibility, balance, and agility to help prevent injuries. To reduce the risk of exercise-related injuries, warm up by performing the exercise at a slow pace before increasing intensity is smart at any age. Take several slow, easy swings of the golf club before teeing off, for example, or cycle at a slow pace to get your muscles ready for a more intense ride. Exercise classes designed for 50+ adults take warm-up and cooldown periods seriously to prevent injury. Also, stay hydrated by drinking cool fluids before, during, and after exercise. In hot, humid summer weather, pay special attention to hydration to avoid heat illness and perform at your best.

MYTH: I can't exercise when I have an injury, such as tennis elbow or an achy knee.

REALITY: Maintaining a schedule of regular physical activity can still be accomplished while nursing minor injuries. You may have to reduce the intensity of your activity and find alternative ways to stay active to prevent aggravation of the injury, but that can and should be done.

MYTH: Red wine is the healthiest of all alcoholic beverages.

REALITY: Red wine contains more phytonutrients than other alcoholic beverages. People often talk about the French diet, which includes red wine, and point out that the French appear to be healthier than Americans despite the fact that their diet includes unhealthy fats. This is known as the French paradox. However, some researchers think it is the red wine the French drink that confers benefit. Wine is part of the typical French meal, which is consumed at a leisurely pace, with wine sipped over several hours. The French don't drink a pitcher of margaritas while eating fried chips and cheese dip. So if you enjoy beer, wine, or spirits, do so in moderation and for social reasons, but don't think of red wine as health food.

Commonly Asked Questions About Chronic Diseases

If partially hydrogenated oil is in the ingredient list of a food, how can the food label state that it has no *trans* fat?

The current labeling laws say that if a food contains less than half a gram of *trans* fat per serving, it can be labeled as having zero grams of *trans* fat. If you eat more than one standard serving, you could be getting more *trans* fats than you think—another good reason to watch portion sizes.

Are organic foods best for treating or preventing cancer?

According to the American Cancer Society, there is no evidence that organic foods are better than conventionally grown foods at reducing cancer risk or improving health outcomes after cancer. The best advice is to eat a variety of whole fruits and vegetables and to wash all vegetables, conventional and organic, in running water to remove any dirt that might have come from the fields or orchards. While there are scary headlines about pesticide residues on foods, "Most scientists and health experts overwhelmingly agree that the mere presence of pesticide residues on food does not mean they are harmful, and that fruits and vegetables grown either conventionally or organically are safe to eat," according to Michael Holsapple, PhD, professor of nutrition and food safety expert at Michigan State University. He goes on to explain that "...for every chemical, including both conventional and organic pesticides, there is a point, or a dose level, that will not produce a harmful response in a living organism. In the world of pesticide regulation, that point is called the No Observed Adverse Effect Level (NOAEL)." To illustrate, he says, "A woman could consume 774 servings of spinach in one day without any effect, even if the spinach had the highest pesticide residues recorded for spinach by the USDA." The bottom line is: Don't let fears of pesticide residues scare you into not eating fruits and vegetables!

Should I choose foods labeled as non-GMO for good health?

This is a personal and polarizing issue for many individuals. First, let's be clear: GMO (short for "genetically modified organism") is not a food but a method, also called genetic engineering, used to enhance or alter the traits of a food. There is no scientific evidence that current genetically engineered crops are harmful to human health. This is based on the conclusions of multiple agencies, including the National Academy of Sciences, the US Department of Agriculture, and the European Food Safety Authority. In fact, there are important benefits to farmers and the environment. For example, genetically engineered corn and cotton are naturally resistant to certain pests, reducing the need for pesticide use. At the time of this writing, the following crops are approved to be genetically modified or genetically engineered: apples, corn, cotton, soybeans, rapeseed (canola), alfalfa, papaya, squash, and sugar beets. The Arctic Apple, a nonbrowning apple, is the newest entry into this category. The Artcic Apple doesn't contain any new genes; rather, scientists found a way to turn off the gene that makes apples brown when cut or sliced and exposed to air. This trait is designed to maintain quality and reduce food waste.

It is important to note that genetically modified wheat is not approved in the United States, so claims that a product is made from wheat that is GMO-free are misleading. Laws require that genetically engineered foods be labeled, and, in the end, it comes down to personal choice. For now, foods certified as 100% organic are GMO-free, so if after you learn more about genetic engineering, you decide you want GMO-free foods, you have that option. One word of caution: if you rely on GMO-free labeling, such as be choosing only non-GMO snack foods, cookies, and candy, you may not be doing your health any favors in the long run. A nutrient-poor food isn't made healthier with a non-GMO label. Our opinion is that GMOs are safe to eat based on current, sound science. Find more information on GMOs in the Useful Resources section on page 284.

How should I choose a fish oil supplement?

Look for a supplement that shows the amount of the omega-3 fats, DHA and EPA, it contains a supplement that says it has 1,200 milligrams of fish oil without showing the actual amount of DHA and EPA may not give you much of either. Recommendations from various health organizations suggest that healthy adults should aim for 250 to 500 milligrams a day of DHA and EPA, so check your supplement labels. Read more about omega-3 fats in Chapter 2.

Is krill oil a good substitute for fish oil?

Krill are tiny crustaceans that are food for many sea creatures. Krill oil can be substituted for fish oil because it contains both DHA and EPA. More research has been conducted with fish oil than with krill oil, but there is no reason to think that krill oil won't improve your blood levels of omega-3 fats. Krill oil capsules are usually smaller than fish oil capsules, and that is a plus for those who have trouble swallowing pills. The downside is they are usually more expensive and usually contain smaller amounts of DHA and EPA.

I don't like fatty fish, but I eat tilapia a couple of times a week. Is that giving me enough omega-3s?

Unfortunately, no. A 4-ounce portion of cooked tilapia has about 150 milligrams of EPA and DHA. Compare that to 4 ounces of farmed Atlantic salmon, which has about 2,400 milligrams of omega-3 fatty acids.

Having the Confidence to Make Food and Fitness Work for You

Whether you plan to totally overhaul your food choices and join a gym tomorrow or if you prefer a small-steps approach, there is no best way to take control of food and fitness after you've been diagnosed with a chronic condition. The most important thing is to realize that striving to be your healthiest at any age is what matters. Don't let a downhill slide become a free fall into losing your health and independence.

A good place to start evaluating your food choices is by doing a pantry/fridge/freezer assessment. While there are about 42,000 foods in a typical grocery store, many of us buy the same items and cook the same meals, time and time again. Take stock of what you have on hand and plan meals with one of the healthy eating plans discussed in Chapter 2. For example, we are guessing that many people have a box of oatmeal in their pantry or cupboard. Of course, oatmeal makes a hearty breakfast by itself, or you can use it to make a healthy granola with chopped nuts, a dash of cinnamon, and a bit of maple syrup to hold it together. Try making oatmeal raisin cookies, or pulse oatmeal in the food processor for a coating for chicken or fish.

Hundreds of recipe websites offer creative ideas for healthy cooking. Following are just a few sites that we like:

- Allrecipes (http://allrecipes.com/recipes/84/healthy-recipes)
- *Cooking Light* magazine (www.cookinglight.com)
- *Eating Well* magazine (www.eatingwell.com)
- Ellie Krieger (www.elliekrieger.com/recipes)
- *Food & Nutrition* magazine (www.foodandnutrition.org)
- Recipe Redux (http://thereciperedux.com)

You might also consider trying a home-delivery meal kit. With these programs, all of the ingredients for a delicious meal are delivered to your door, complete with step-by-step instructions to get dinner on the table in about 30 minutes.

Another good strategy is to use the information provided throughout the book to make small changes to boost nutrient intake. While tracking calories on a smartphone app is useful, it doesn't tell you much about the quality of your diet. Using the example of calcium, the table on page 280 gives examples of small changes the can be made to each meal and snack to meet daily calcium needs.

Conversation with an Expert

John Davis Cantwell, MD, MACP, FACC, is now in his mid-70s and still has a thriving practice as a cardiologist at the Piedmont Heart Institute in Atlanta, Georgia. He is also a team physician for the Atlanta Braves and the team cardiologist for the athletes at Georgia Tech. In 1996, he was the chief medical officer for the Atlanta Olympic Games. John was an early adopter of preventive medicine. He recalls, "My clinical research focused on preventive cardiology, cardiac rehabilitation, and sports cardiology. It has been rewarding to see all three areas emerge into mainstream medicine, compared to when my practice began in 1972."

From an early age, as a three-sport high school athlete and a two-sport athlete at Duke University, physical activity was just part of John's daily life. He says:

> In medical school, I began to run a mile most days on the cinder track adjacent to the school to maintain some level of fitness. For many years afterward, my wife and

SIMPLE CHANGES TO BOOST CALCIUM TO MEET THE NEEDS OF A 70+ WOMAN (target of 1,200 milligrams of calcium)

USUAL INTAKE	Calcium (milligrams)	Meal/ Snack Total Calcium (milligrams)	BOOSTED INTAKE	Calcium (milligrams)	Meal/ Snack Total Calcium (milligrams)
Breakfast					
Coffee, black	5		Latte coffee with milk	138	
Instant oatmeal	104		Oatmeal with toppings:	104	
			1 ounce chopped almonds	76	
Banana	5	**114**	1 ounce berries	9	**327**
Lunch					
Chicken noodle soup	7		6 ounces vanilla yogurt with toppings :	258	
Snack crackers	25		homemade granola with almonds	40	
Handful peanuts	20				
Sliced apple	7	**59**	Whole orange	70	**368**
Snack					
Pretzel sticks	0	**0**	Handful peanuts	20	**20**
Dinner					
Grilled steak	0		Grilled turkey burger with Swiss cheese	240	
Caesar salad	60		Wilted spinach salad	145	
Baked potato with skin	20		Parmesan roasted potatoes	200	
Steamed carrots	35				
Iced tea	0	**115**	Iced tea	0	**585**
Snack					
Chocolate chip cookies	0	**0**	Italian ice	100	**100**
Totals		**288**			**1,688**

> I would run five miles most days. I found this a good way to dissipate stress and to maintain my weight and blood pressure, and I also noted that it helped me to formulate ideas for my writing and public speaking.

In hindsight, he wishes he had done more cross-training, "...like my sister-in-law, who continues at age 70 to do aerobics, golf, and tennis without excessive strain on her joints." He and his wife both sport two artificial hips, a testament to years of wear and tear from running. However, that only made him alter his fitness routine. He explains, "At present, we try to do an hour of walking or one-speed biking most days, and I add some aerobic weight training for muscle toning."

His diet typifies what we have been advocating in the pages of this book. He says:

> I try to eat prudently without being a dietary fanatic. We try to limit red meat, fast foods, and excessive simple carbohydrates and emphasize vegetables, fruits, and fish, such as salmon. As a youth, I probably consumed too many hamburgers and french fries and malted milks!

Today, his biggest challenge is eating fewer cookies and steering clear of "the mint ice cream sandwiches in the Braves' visiting team's locker room."

John says, "Now, at age 76, I agree with Ken Cooper [PhD] who said, 'We are all going to die of something, just don't die of something stupid.'" Doing "something stupid" includes binge alcohol drinking, smoking, not paying attention to your numbers (blood pressure, blood fats), drug abuse, and not keeping up with prudent preventive screening, such as mammograms, colonoscopies, and prostate examinations. He also recommends that "one should seek help for symptoms of depression, which can increase the risk of suicide if untreated, and avoid excessive sun exposure to reduce the risk of skin cancer."

Here are John's goals for his patients:

1. Strive to get your body mass index below 25 with a healthy diet and daily exercise.

2. Get a home blood pressure kit and aim to keep readings below 140/90, ideally 120/80.

3. Get a coronary calcium scan for men beginning at age 40 and for women at age 50. Those with any significant calcium scores should aim to bring low-density lipoprotein cholesterol levels under 70 in order to stabilize coronary plaque development. Follow a diet low in saturated fats, and use statin drugs when necessary.

4. Women of all ages and men age 65 and older should consume no more than one standard-sized alcoholic drink in a day and should avoid alcohol altogether if there is any family history of alcoholism.

5. Try to average 10,000 steps of exercise most days, and avoid prolonged sitting.

John agrees with Henry David Thoreau, who wrote, "We are all builders of a temple, called (our) body.... we are all sculptors and painters, and our material is our own flesh and blood and bones." His goal as a physician is to "help patients become better temple builders."

How the Authors Try to Combat Chronic Diseases

Both Chris and Bob have experienced bad stuff as they have aged, as illustrated in their personal stories in this chapter. Here is what they did when bad stuff happened and how they try to keep chronic diseases at bay.

Chris: In addition to hip surgery and breast cancer, I had rotator cuff repair surgery several years ago. After every injury or illness, I have found ways to adapt and strive for good health. When it comes to exercise, I had to change my routine to find new ways to be active every day. I gave up running after my hip replacement but found enjoyment in cycling and aerobic dance classes. Yoga has helped strengthen my hip and shoulder muscles, although I still find push-ups a challenge! Using a fitness tracker helps me monitor activities and is a visual reminder to get up and move throughout the day, every day. And I walk with two big dogs every day. I am a big believer in preventive screenings and vaccines, and I keep up with these preventive measures as recommended by my doctor. I know that these won't prevent me from ever getting sick, but they do decrease the odds, and that is a good reason to keep up with screenings and vaccines. I monitor my blood lipids for the usual cholesterol and triglycerides, but I also have my omega-3 index measured to learn whether my supplement strategy is working to keep my omega-3 levels in a healthy range.

Bob: Aside from spending three decades trying to get my atrial fibrillation under control, I've been very fortunate not to have any chronic diseases—as of my late 60s, anyway. I try my best to lead a healthy lifestyle and keep my diet, fitness routine, and health behaviors from becoming too extreme. I exercise more than most people my age but try not to allow my devotion to staying active interfere with social activities or time with my wife. My diet is on the healthy side, but not to any extremes in terms of counting calories, taking special supplements, or depriving myself of enjoyable foods and snacks. I keep annual appointments with my cardiologist and primary-care physician, along with regular visits with the dentist, to make sure that I'm staying on top of potential problems. I haven't been good about getting an annual flu shot, so that's something for me to consider. My body weight and body mass index are normal for my height, and I don't have any nagging joint issues that limit my movements. My wristwatch is set to remind me to take at least a few minute-long breaks each hour that I'm working in the office or in front of the television to ensure that I don't spend too much time sitting. I'm well aware that good health is not a guarantee, and I'm trying to take care of myself in all the right ways so that I can continue to enjoy an active and fun life with friends and loved ones for decades to come.

Useful Resources

American Diabetes Association (www.diabetes.org/food-and-fitness)
▷ *Using food and fitness to prevent and treat diabetes*

American Heart Association (www.heart.org/HEARTORG/Conditions/Conditions_UCM_001087_SubHomePage.jsp)
▷ *Information on all aspects of heart disease, including high blood pressure, stroke, peripheral vascular disease, congestive heart failure, and coronary heart disease*

Arthritis Foundation (www.arthritis.org/about-arthritis)
▷ *Resources for dealing with arthritis*

Center for Science in the Public Interest (https://cspinet.org/protecting-our-health/biotechnology)
▷ *Information on biotechnology and health*

Centers for Disease Control and Prevention (www.cdc.gov/tobacco/data_statistics/fact_sheets/cessation/quitting/index.htm and www.cdc.gov/tobacco/data_statistics/fact_sheets/tobacco_industry/cigars/index.htm)
▷ *Resources for quitting smoking cigarettes and cigars*

Centers for Disease Control and Prevention (www.cdc.gov/vaccines/vpd/shingles/public/index.html)
▷ *Information about the shingles vaccine*

Council for Biotechnology Information (https://gmoanswers.com)
▷ *Answers to common questions about GMO*

Distilled Spirits Council of the United States (www.drinkinmoderation.org)
▷ *Guidelines for drinking in moderation*

Food and Agriculture Organization of the United Nations, International Year of Pulses 2016 (www.fao.org/pulses-2016/en)
▷ *Information about pulses (beans, peas, and lentils) and recipes*

FoodSafety.gov (www.foodsafety.gov)
▷ *Food safety tips and recalls*

Harvard Health Publications (www.health.harvard.edu/staying-healthy/foods-that-fight-inflammation)
▷ *Food and nutrition resources, including information on foods that fight inflammation*

National Council on Aging (www.ncoa.org/healthy-aging/falls-prevention)
▷ *Fall prevention strategies*

National Heart, Lung, and Blood Institute (www.nhlbi.nih.gov/files/docs/public/heart/hbp_low.pdf)
▷ *Guide to lowering blood pressure*

National Osteoporosis Foundation (www.nof.org/patients/communication-with-your-doctor/doctor-visit-checklist)
▷ *Doctor-visit checklist*

OmegaQuant (www.omegaquant.com)
▷ *Blood testing for omega-3 levels*

EPILOGUE

Old age is the thirst for knowledge.

POPE FRANCIS AT AGE 76, DURING HIS FIRST PAPAL GREETING (2013)

IN THE PREFACE, we introduced you to Stephanie, who wanted to take control of her food and fitness as she approached her 50th birthday. Stephanie's story is one that resonated with us, and we hope it resonated with you, too. It's not uncommon that we put others first. Spouses or partners, children or grandchildren, bosses, work, and community commitments often come before our own health. Many people fall into habits that seem hard to change, but with a bit of planning and the realization that health matters, anyone can make meaningful changes to eat well, move well, and be well at any age. As we've shown you throughout this book, small changes can have big results. Eating one more calcium-rich food a day, consuming more protein at lunch, meeting a friend for a workout, doing some stretching exercises during television commercials, and sticking to a routine for restful sleep can improve the quality, and maybe the quantity, of our lives.

How did Stephanie's journey end? Let's get an update on her goal of being "fit and fifty."

Stephanie's initial success motivated her to get more serious about her quest. She researched several eating plans and settled on a high-protein/moderate-carbohydrate plan that was sustainable for the long haul. She wasn't looking for a no-carb, quick weight loss plan, as she knew she wouldn't be able to stick to a severely restricted diet over time. She also learned that exercise needed to be a key component of her plan to achieve fitness and relieve stress. A fitness tracker seemed like a good way to monitor steps and track calorie expenditure. She admitted that in the early months she was a slave to the tracker; she couldn't go to bed unless she reached the magic number of 10,000 steps. She cultivated a friend as her walking buddy, and they motivated each other to exercise, squeezing in walks whenever they could, whether in the early mornings or late evenings; neither wanted to let the other down. Stephanie also decided to join a gym and take advantage of group classes. Her goal, to lose about 30 pounds before her 50th birthday, was met by sticking with a combination of diet and exercise. Her reward was a stylish, fitted dress for her birthday bash. Stephanie now likes the way she looks in clothes, and she had not felt that way for a long time.

Stephanie faced challenges, as we all do, while undertaking self-improvement. She missed eating some of her favorite foods and found herself cooking different meals for herself and her family. Exercising when she didn't feel like it was a struggle. Making time for exercise required a commitment to set it as a priority.

Stephanie's story didn't end there; like many of us over 50, an injury complicated her plans. She hurt her back and had to substitute physical therapy for regular gym sessions. Coupled with the holiday season and travel, she gained a few pounds. But she is back on track and motivated to pick up where she left off, with newfound persistence and patience to go the distance.

Stephanie's story has all of the elements that inspire us. While diet and exercise sound easy, they are anything but. Who among us wouldn't love to find a magic weight-loss pill or 1-minute exercise (or better yet, exercise in a pill), but in our heart of hearts, we know it takes hard work and dedication. Weight gain after weight loss is common. The key is to monitor your weight and not let a 2-pound weight gain become 20 pounds. The same goes for exercise; everyone will have to miss an exercise class or cancel a planned bike ride every now and then, but getting right back into a routine is what matters. Too many of us say to ourselves, "I'll start eating better on Monday" (usually said on Friday night), or "I'll join a gym on January 2." Better to start now, at the next meal or at the next break in your day when you could fit in movement.

We hope that as you age, your thirst for knowledge to eat healthy and pursue fitness will continue to grow. Aging brings many changes, both positive and negative, and at some point, everyone will need to find a new normal. We hope we have shown you that while there is no one best way to eat or be active, you can improve your food choices, customize a supplement plan, and improve aerobic and muscular fitness at any age.

Earlier in the book, we stressed that while there is no one best eating plan or best exercise routine, it is important to remember that good food and fitness improve many health outcomes. While weight training might improve muscle mass, it also strengthens bones and revs up calorie burning. So remember that you will get multiple benefits from improving your food choices and from getting and staying active.

We want to end by offering you a few more tips for eating well, moving well, and being well.

Eat Well

- Try one new food or recipe each week to challenge your taste buds and break out of a food rut.
- Plan your meals. This saves time and money in the long run.
- Start a supper club with like-minded friends to try healthy recipes and new meal ideas.
- Make vegetables and whole grains the main focus of your plate instead of centering meals on the protein portion.
- Be the one in your family or group of friends who brings healthy appetizers, entrées, sides, or desserts to events, showcasing how nutritious can be delicious.

Move Well

- Keep your walking or running shoes by the door to remind you to be active.
- Improve your grip strength with hand squeeze grippers. Keep them visible and use them several times a day to keep hands and fingers strong.
- Cross-train. Do different types of exercises and challenges your muscles with new routines for the best results.
- Make time for at least 30 minutes of moderate-to-vigorous physical activity each day, even if you have to do it as three 10-minute bouts.

Be Well

- Be an informed consumer of diet, exercise, and health advice. Read beyond the headlines to get the full story; we often find that the latest and greatest health study might have been conducted with mice, not humans.
- Be savvy about internet health searches. Learn to move beyond the first few hits of a search, as many internet links are advertisements designed to get us to purchase a product.
- Use credible sources for health information. Professional organizations, such as the Academy of Nutrition and Dietetics and the American College of Sports Medicine, are good places to start for information on food and fitness. When researching a disease, try a professional organization first to gain a broad understanding of the topic.
- Be wary of any food, exercise, or supplement that claims to be groundbreaking. Science is evolutionary, not revolutionary.

APPENDIX A
DEFINITION OF TERMS

Term	Definition
Aerobic fitness	The capacity to perform extended physical activity
Cardiovascular disease	A group of diseases and disorders affecting the heart and blood vessels, including blocked coronary arteries, electrical abnormalities, and problems with the various heart valves
Cardiovascular fitness	Synonymous with aerobic fitness
Dietary Guidelines for Americans	A set of evidence-based recommendations designed to help Americans eat a healthy diet *The guidelines are updated every 5 years based on a review of current science by an advisory committee of food and nutrition experts. The most recent edition is the 2015-2020* Dietary Guidelines for Americans.
Eating plan	A system for eating; also called food pattern or dietary pattern *Throughout this book, we use the term "healthy eating plan" to describe the plans we think are best for older adults.*
Essential body fat	The amount of stored body fat needed for good health and normal functioning *For men, essential body fat percentage is about 5%, and for women, it is about 12%; this is not considered a desirable percentage of body fat but simply the minimal amount needed for good health.*
Gastric reflux	A condition when the stomach contents, which are normally acidic, splash up into the lower part of the esophagus (the tube that runs from your throat to the stomach) and causes a burning pain in the middle of the chest
Glucagon	A hormone made by the pancreas that helps increase blood sugar when it gets too low, such as after an overnight fast before you have eaten breakfast
Hormone	A naturally occurring chemical produced in the body that is carried through the blood and has a specific effect on regulating a body function *For example, the hormone insulin is made in the pancrease but acts on muscle, fat, and liver cells by allowing blood sugar to enter those tissues so that it can be used for energy or storage.*

Insulin	A hormone made in the pancreas that is released into the blood after eating to help lower blood sugar when it gets too high
Lipid profile	A panel of blood tests that measures blood cholesterol, triglycerides, and particles (lipoproteins, such as low-density lipoproteins [LDLs] and high-density lipoprotein [HDLs]) that carry the fats through the blood
Metabolic syndrome	A group of three or more factors (such as high blood pressure, excess belly fat, high triglyceride levels, low HDL levels, and high blood sugar levels) that are linked to an increased risk of cardiovascular disease and type 2 diabetes *This is also called insulin resistance syndrome and was originally known as "syndrome X"*
Moderate-intensity exercise	Physical activity conducted at a pace that allows for talking but not singing *Examples include walking faster than a 20-minute mile or bicycling slower than 10 mph.*
Progressive resistance exercise	Strength-training exercise that uses weights, elastic bands/straps, machines, or body weight to gradually increase muscle strength over a period of months
Type 1 diabetes	A disorder where the pancreas stops making any insulin, resulting in the need to take insulin shots for survival *Only about 5% of diabetes cases are type 1.*
Type 2 diabetes	The most common form of diabetes *This is a chronic and progressive condition that affects the body's ability to control blood sugar levels.*
VO_2 max	A laboratory measurement of maximal aerobic fitness *Commonly performed on a treadmill or stationary bicycle, this test requires an all-out maximal effort to exhaustion. Other tests estimate VO_2 max from submaximal exercise.*

APPENDIX B
POPULAR DIETARY SUPPLEMENTS USED IN THE MANAGEMENT OF CHRONIC DISEASES

Supplement	What Is It, and Why Is It Used?	Is It Effective?	Things to Consider
Alpha-lipoic acid	Antioxidant used for diabetes and diabetic neuropathy (nerve pain)	Possibly helpful for decreasing blood sugar, though not all studies show that it lowers blood sugar Improves symptoms of diabetic nerve pain in some people	People with diabetes should check blood sugar levels; the combination of alpha-lipoic acid and diabetes medicines might cause hypoglycemia (low blood sugar). Never stop taking diabetes medicine without talking to your doctor. Don't take this supplement if you take thyroid medicine; it can reduce the effectiveness of the thyroid drug.
Calcium	The most abundant mineral in the body; needed for bone health and for muscle and blood vessel contraction and relaxation, nerve transmission, and hormone secretion	Can help you reach the recommended amount	Calcium citrate is the recommended form of calcium for adults age 50 and over. Calcium citrate does not need stomach acid for absorption, so it can be taken with or without food. It is best absorbed in doses of 500 milligrams or less, so divide doses throughout the day.
Citicoline	A compound used in brain cell membranes and to make the chemical-signaling molecules in the brain	Possibly effective for age-related memory problems and recovery from stroke	It is safe in doses of 250–500 milligrams, although research studies use higher doses of 1,000–2,000 milligrams a day. There are no known drug interactions, but always tell your doctor about supplements you are taking.

Supplement	What Is It, and Why Is It Used?	Is It Effective?	Things to Consider
Coenzyme Q10	Vitamin-like compound found in many organs (heart, liver, kidney) used to treat heart diseases, diseases of blood vessels, diabetic neuropathy, high blood pressure, and migraine headaches; may also be used for muscle pain by people taking statin drugs to lower cholesterol	Possibly helpful for the conditions mentioned but should not replace medicines used to treat the diseases; seems to be more effective when taken with prescribed drugs Possibly effective at treating muscle pain from statin drugs (some studies show a positive effect and others show no effect) Claims to improve athletic performance, but does not improve endurance or strength exercises	It can cause mild gastrointestinal side effects, but taking smaller doses several times a day might help. Monitoring blood pressure is necessary. It may interfere with blood clotting medicines (Coumadin).
Fiber	Psyllium and methycelluose (the most common fiber supplements)	Possibly helpful for lowering cholesterol and blood sugar Claims to increase fullness for weight management	Fiber supplements can cause gas and bloating, especially when going from a low fiber intake to a high fiber intake without taking time for the body to adjust. Fiber supplements don't provide the nutrients that fruits, vegetables, or whole grains do. Drink an 8-ounce glass of water with each dose. Tell your doctor about fiber supplements, as they may interfere with absorption of some prescription medicines.

Supplement	What Is It, and Why Is It Used?	Is It Effective?	Things to Consider
Flax seed oil	Contains the essential fatty acid alpha-linolenic acid (ALA)	Many claims are made for use, but best for getting ALA (it is has the highest concentration of ALA of any plant) Not a substitute for fish oils (eicosapentaenoic acid [EPA] and docosahexaenoic acid [DHA]); only 5% to 10% of ALA is converted to EPA and DHA	The usual dose is 1 or 2 tablespoons a day. ALA is destroyed by heat, so flax seed oil should not be used for cooking.
Glucosamine and chondroitin	Substances found in cartilage, a connective tissue that covers the ends of bones where joints are formed	May relieve knee and hip pain in those with osteoarthritis at doses of 1,500 milligrams of glucosamine and 1,200 milligrams of chondroitin	If pain relief does not occur within 3 months, discontinue use. Glucosamine may affect eye pressure, so talk to your doctor if you are being treated for glaucoma. Most supplements are made from shrimp or crab shells, so if you are allergic to seafood, find a supplement made from other ingredients.
Hibiscus tea	A red flowering plant used to make tea, jam, sauces, and flavoring for other foods	Possibly effective for lowering blood pressure when used for 2–6 weeks	If you are on blood pressure-lowering medications, talk to your doctor before taking this supplement, and monitor your pressure so it doesn't go too low.
Multivitamin	A pill, capsule, or chewable that provides most essential nutrients	Can fill nutrient gaps but cannot provide 100% of the Recommended Dietary Allowances for all nutrients	Choose a multivitamin and mineral supplement designed for adults age 50 and over. Look for third-party verification, like the initials USP (US Pharmacopoeia), to ensure that the supplement is of high quality. More isn't better; take only the recommended dose. Take with food.

Supplement	What Is It, and Why Is It Used?	Is It Effective?	Things to Consider
Omega-3 fatty acids (fish oil)	Two long-chain polyunsaturated fats, EPA and DHA, which are found in fatty fish, like salmon, mackerel, and tuna, and in fish oil supplements	Can lower cholesterol and fight inflammation Can reduce the stickiness of platelets that contribute to blood clotting	Keep doses under 2 grams a day. Enteric-coated fish oil capsules reduce "fish burps," a common complaint of those who take fish oil.
Turmeric	Spice used in many cuisines, especially curry; active compound is curcumin, which gives curry and mustard a yellow-orange color An antioxidant and anti-inflammatory spice	Has been used to reduce inflammation in both patients with rheumatoid arthritis, osteoarthritis, and other inflammatory conditions, such as irritable bowel syndrome	Dietary intake is around 60–100 milligrams a day for those who eat curry, but research studies with turmeric use much higher doses: 1,000–1,500 milligrams or more a day. Turmeric is better absorbed with foods or meals that contain fat.
Vitamin D	Fat-soluble vitamin needed to help absorb calcium in the gut; also used for bone growth; regulating cell growth; nerve, muscle, and immune function; and reducing inflammation	Can elevate blood levels in those who are deficient or who have less than optimal levels	Both vitamins D-2 and D-3 are effective for raising blood levels, but D-3 is slightly more potent. More isn't better; the upper tolerable limit is 4,000 International Units a day. Therapeutic intakes may be higher but should only be taken under a doctor's supervision.

Sources:

Natural Medicines Comprehensive Database, http://naturaldatabase.therapeuticresearch.com/home.aspx?cs=&s=ND

ConsumerLab: www.consumerlab.com/

National Institutes of Health, Office of Dietary Supplements, https://ods.od.nih.gov/

National Institutes of Health, National Center for Complementary and Integrative Health: https://nccih.nih.gov/

APPENDIX C
PROTEIN-RICH FOODS AND POWDERS

Food	Protein Classification	Portion Size for 25 g of Protein	Notes
Milk	Complete protein Contains 2 protein fractions: whey and casein	3 cups (24 ounces)	The combination of whey and casein makes milk a great food for muscle building and recovery after exercise. You can find milk with added protein, either through fortification or special filtration to concentrate protein. Milk naturally contains the sugar lactose, which some people can't tolerate, but there are many lactose-free options.
Yogurt	Complete protein Greek-yogurt contains more protein than traditional yogurt	1 cup (8 ounces) for Greek-yogurt 3 cups (24 ounces) for traditional yogurt	Yogurt can be a good source of probiotics to support gut health.
Eggs	Complete protein Often said to be the gold standard for protein quality	3 large whole eggs 7 large egg whites	Most of the protein is found in the yolk.
Beef	Complete protein	3 ounces, cooked	Beef is also a good source of the minerals and vitamins needed as we age. Choose lean cuts more often.
Poultry	Complete protein	3 ounces, cooked	Dark meat has more minerals than white meat.
Pork	Complete protein	3 ounces, cooked	Although it is pork, bacon is mostly fat and has less than 3 grams of protein per slice. Choose lean cuts more often.

Food	Protein Classification	Portion Size for 25 g of Protein	Notes
Fish/ Seafood	Complete protein	3 ounces cooked fish 5 ounces cooked shrimp, scallops, or lobster 1 crab leg	Fatty fish provide omega-3 fatty acids.
Soy	Complete protein	3 (8-ounces) cups soy milk 4 slices firm tofu 1 cup edamame 2 soy burgers	Soy protein is a good choice for vegetarians or for those who want to eat less meat yet consume quality protein.
Nuts	Incomplete protein	4 ounces (92 almonds) 6 ounces (108 cashews) 4 ounces (196 pistachios) 6 ounces (84 halves) walnuts 3.5 ounces (40 peanuts)	Nuts are a tasty way to increase protein and healthy fats, but they are also high in calories. Use nuts as an ingredient in a dish or as a topping on salads, fruit, or yogurt. Eat smaller portions for a snack.
Pea protein	Incomplete protein	1 scoop* (about 3 tablespoons)	This powder, made from yellow peas, is a good choice for those with soy allergies.
Chia seeds	Incomplete protein	1 ounce (2 tablespoons)	Chia seeds have high antioxidant activity and supply fiber.
Hemp protein	Incomplete protein	2 scoops* (about 6 tablespoons)	This emerging protein source is from the same plant as marijuana, but a different variety, so it should contain only trace amounts of tetrahydrocannabinol.
Whey protein	Complete protein	1 scoop* (about 3 tablespoons)	Whey, the liquid portion left over from making cheese, is the most well researched of all proteins for muscle building and recovery after exercise. It is most often sold as a powdered product.

*Most protein powers contain 15 to 30 grams of protein per 33-gram scoop, but check the label to be sure.

BIBLIOGRAPHY

Chapter 1

Amati F, Dubé JJ, Coen DM, Stefanvic-Racic M, Toledo FG, Goodpaster BH. Physical inactivity and obesity underlie the insulin resistance of aging. *Diabetes Care*. 2009;32(8):1547-1549.

Clarke TC, Ward BW, Freeman G, Schiller JS. Early release of selected estimates based on data from the January–September 2015 National Health Interview Survey. National Center for Health Statistics. www.cdc.gov/nchs/data/nhis/earlyrelease/earlyrelease201602.pdf. Published February 2016. Accessed March 26, 2017.

Facts about physical activity. May 23, 2014. Centers for Disease Control and Prevention website. www.cdc.gov/physicalactivity/data/facts.htm. Updated May 23, 2015. Accessed April 1, 2017.

Fiatarone MA, O'Neill EF, Ryan ND, et al. Exercise training and nutritional supplementation for physical frailty in very elderly people. *N Engl J Med*.1994;330:1769-1775.

Food Insight. 2016 Food and Health Survey: "Food Decision 2016: The Impact of a Growing National Food Dialogue." International Food Information Council Foundation website. www.foodinsight.org/articles/2016-food-and-health-survey-food-decision-2016-impact-growing-national-food-dialogue. Updated October 14, 2016. Accessed March 23, 2017.

Health and Retirement: Planning for the great unknown. A Merrill Lynch retirement study conducted in partnership with Age Wave. 2015. Age Wave website. http://agewave.com/what-we-do/landmark-research-and-consulting/research-studies/health-and-retirement-planning-for-the-great-unknown/.Published 2015. Accessed April 5, 2017.

Janssen I. Sarcopenia. In: Bales CW, Ritchie, CS, eds. *Handbook of Clinical Nutrition and Aging*. 2nd ed, New York: Humana Press, New York; 2009:183-205.

Khera AV, Emdin CA, Drake I, et al. Genetic risk, adherence to a healthy lifestyle, and coronary disease. *N Engl J Med*. 2016;375(24):2349-2358. www.nejm.org/doi/full/10.1056/NEJMoa1605086#t=article.

Maron BJ, Araújo CGS, Thompson PD, et al. Recommendations for preparticipation screening and the assessment of cardiovascular disease in masters athletes. *Circulation*. 2001:103:327-334.

Produce for Better Health Foundation. State of the Plate: 2015 Study on America's Consumption of Fruit and Vegetables. Hockessin, DE: Produce for Better Health Foundation; 2015. www.pbhfoundation.org/pdfs/about/res/pbh_res/State_of_the_Plate_2015_WEB_Bookmarked.pdf.

Sallinen,J, Ojanen T, Karavirta L, Ahtiainen JP, Häkkinen K. Muscle mass and strength, body composition and dietary intake in master strength athletes vs untrained men of different ages. *J Sports Med Phys Fitness*. 2008;48(2):190-196.

Talking with patients about weight loss: tips for primary care providers. National Institute of Diabetes and Digestive and Kidney Diseases website. www.niddk.nih.gov/health-information/health-topics/weight-control/talking-with-patients-about-weight-loss-tips-for-primary-care/Pages/talking.aspx#j. Published January 2017. Accessed March 2, 2017.

Tanaka H, Seals DR. Endurance exercise performance in Masters athletes: age-associated changes and underlying physiological mechanisms. *J Physiol.* 2009;586(1):55-63.

Wright VJ, Perricelli BC. Age-related rates of decline in performance among elite senior athletes. *Am J Sports Med.* 2008;36(3):443-450.

Chapter 2

Anderson JJ, Nieman DC. Diet quality—the Greeks had it right. *Nutrients.* 2016;8(10):piiE636.

Fitch C, Keim KS, Academy of Nutrition and Dietetics. Position of the Academy of Nutrition and Dietetics: use ofnutritive and nonnutritive sweeteners. *J Acad Nutr Diet.* 2012;112(8):739-758.

Freedland-Graves JH, Nitzke S, Academy of Nutrition and Dietetics. Position of the Academy of Nutrition and Dietetics: total diet approach to healthy eating. *J Acad Nutr Diet.* 2013;113(2):307-317.

Frieden TR. Sodium reduction—saving lives by putting choice into consumers' hands. *JAMA.* 2016;316(6):579-580.

Hodge AM, O'Dea K, English DR, Giles GG, Flicker L. Dietary patterns as predictors of successful ageing. *J Nutr Health Aging.* 2014;18(3):221-227.

Jiang R, Jacobs DR Jr, Mayer-Davis E, et al. Nut and seed consumption and inflammatory markers in the multi-ethnic study of atherosclerosis. *Am J Epidemiol.* 2006;163(3):222–231. doi:10.1093/aje/kwj033.

Koch M, Jensen MK. Association of the MIND diet with cognition and risk of Alzheimer's disease. *Curr Opin Lipidol.* 2016;27(3):303-304.

Martínez-González MA. Benefits of the Mediterranean diet beyond the Mediterranean Sea and beyond food patterns. *BMC Med.* 2016;14:157.

Martínez-González MA, Salas-Salvadó J, Estruch R, et al. Benefits of the Mediterranean diet: insights from the PREDIMED study. *Prog Cardiovasc Dis.* 2015;58(1):50-60. doi: 10.1016/j.pcad.2015.04.003.

Melina V, Craig W, Levin S. Position of the Academy of Nutrition and Dietetics: vegetarian diets. *J Acad Nutr Diet.* 2016;116(12):1970-1980.

Ndanuko RN, Tapsell LC, Charlton KE, Neale EP, Batterham MJ. Dietary patterns and blood pressure in adults: a systematic review and meta-analysis of randomized controlled trials. *Adv Nutr.* 2016;7(1):76-89.

Slawson DL, Fitzgerald N, Morgan KT. Position of the Academy of Nutrition and Dietetics: the role of nutrition in health promotion and chronic disease prevention. *J Acad Nutr Diet.* 2013;113(7):972-979.

Tangney CC, Li H,Wang Y, et al. Relation of DASH- and Mediterranean-like dietary patterns to cognitive decline in older persons. *Neurology.* 2014;83(16):1410-1416.

Tapsell LC, Neale EP, Satija A, Hu FB. Foods, nutrients, and dietary patterns: interconnections and implications for dietary guidelines. *Adv Nutr.* 2016;7:445-454.

US Department of Health and Human Services and US Department of Agriculture. *2015–2020 Dietary Guidelines for Americans*. 8th ed. December 2015. http://health.gov/dietaryguidelines/2015/guidelines/. Published December 2015.

Chapter 3

American College of Sports Medicine, Sawka MN, Burke LM, et al. American College of Sports Medicine position stand. Exercise and fluid replacement. *Med Sci Sports Exerc*. 2007;39(2):377-390.

Institute of Medicine. *Dietary Reference Intakes for Water, Potassium, Sodium, Chloride, and Sulfate*. Washington, DC: National Academies Press; 2005.

Murray B. Fluid, electrolytes, and exercise. In: Rosenbloom CA, Coleman EJ, eds. *Sports Nutrition: A Practice Manual for Professionals*, 5th ed. Chicago: Academy of Nutrition and Dietetics; 2012.

Valtin H. "Drink at least eight glasses of water a day." Really? Is there scientific evidence for "8 x 8"? *Am J Physiol Regul Integr Comp Physiol*. 2002;283(5):R993-R1004.

Chapter 4

Erdman JW Jr, Smith JW, Kuchan MJ, et al. Lutein and brain function. *Foods*. 2015.4(4):547-564. doi:10.3390/foods4040547.

Firnhaber JM, Kolasa KM. Harden my heart: calcium supplementation and the risk of cardiovascular disease risk. *Nutr Today*. 2016;51(1):18-24.

Ghezzi P, Jaquet V, Marcucci F, Schmidt HH. The oxidative stress theory of disease: levels of evidence and epistemological aspects. *Br J Pharmacol*. 2016 Jul 18. doi: 10.1111/bph.13544. Epub ahead of print.

Hooshmand B, Mangialasche F, Kalpouzos G, et al. Association of vitamin B12, folate, and sulfur amino acids with brain magnetic resonance imaging measures in older adults: a longitudinal population-based study. *JAMA Psychiatry*. 2016;73(6):606-613. doi:10.1001/jamapsychiatry.2016.0274.

Institute of Medicine; Otten JJ, Hellwig JP, Meyers LD, eds. *Dietary Reference Intakes: The Essential Guide to Nutrient Requirements*. 2006. Washington, DC: National Academies Press; 2006.

Kumar S, Pandey AK. Chemistry and biological activities of flavonoids: an overview. *Sci World J*. 2013;2013:1-16.

McCullough ML, Peterson JJ, Patel R, Jacques PF, Shah R. Dwyer JT. Flavonoid intake and cardiovascular disease mortality in a prospective cohort of US adults. *Am J Clin Nutr*. 2012;95(2):454-464.

US Department of Agriculture, Bhagwat S, Haytowitz DB. USDA Database for the Flavonoid Content of Selected Foods. Release 3.2. US Department of Agriculture, Agricultural Research Service. www.ars.usda.gov/nutrientdata/flav. Updated November 2015. Accessed July 7, 2017.

Wang X, Ouyang Y, Liu J, et al. Fruit and vegetable consumption and mortality from all causes, cardiovascular disease, and cancer: systematic review and dose-response meta-analysis of prospective cohort studies. *BMJ*. 2014;349:g4490. doi: 10.1136/bmj.g4490.

What are Phytohnutrients? Fruits and Veggies More Matters website. www.fruitsandveggiesmorematters.org/what-are-phytochemicals. Accessed July 7, 2017.

Chapter 5

Goodman JM, Burr JF, Banks L, Thomas SG. The acute risks of exercise in apparently healthy adults and relevance for prevention of cardiovascular events. *Can J Cardiol.* 2016;32(4):523-532.

Han TS, Lean ME. A clinical perspective of obesity, metabolic syndrome and cardiovascular disease. *JRSM Cardiovasc Dis.* 2016;5:2048004016633371. doi: 10.1177/2048004016633371.

He W, Goodkind D, Kowai P. An Aging World: 2015, US Census Bureau. www.census.gov/content/dam/Census/library/publications/2016/demo/p95-16-1.pdf. Published March 2016. Accessed March 29, 2017.

Joyner MJ, Landman N, Smoldt RK, White AR, Cortese DE. A Roadmap to Better Health. CreateSpace Independent Publishing Platform website; 2015. https://marketplace.cms.gov/outreach-and-education/downloads/c2c-roadmap.pdf Accessed April 5, 2017.

Shephard RJ. Aging and Exercise. In: Fahey TD, ed. *Encyclopedia of Sports Medicine and Science.* internet Society for Sport Science website. www.sportsci.org/encyc/agingex/agingex.html. Published March 7, 1998. Accessed December 21, 2016.

Song M, Giovannucci E. Preventable incidence and mortality of carcinoma associated with lifestyle factors among white adults in the United States. *JAMA Oncol.* 2016;2(9):1154-1161. doi:10.1001/jamaoncol.2016.0843.

Watson KB, Carlson SA, Gunn JP, et al. Physical inactivity among adults aged 50 years and older—United States, 2014. *MMWR Morb Mortal Wkly Rep.* 2016;65:954–958. doi: http://dx.doi.org/10.15585/mmwr.mm6536a3.

Chapter 6

Crane JD, Macneil LG, Tarnopolsky MAl. Long-term aerobic exercise is associated with greater muscle strength throughout the life span. *J Gerontol A Biol Sci Med Sci.* 2013;68(6):631-638, 2013.

Shephard RJ. Aging and Exercise. In: Fahey TD, ed. *Encyclopedia of Sports Medicine and Science.* internet Society for Sport Science website. www.sportsci.org/encyc/agingex/agingex.html. Published March 7, 1998. Accessed December 21, 2016.

Witard OC, McGlory C, Hamilton DL, Phillips SM. Growing older with health and vitality: a nexus of physical activity, exercise and nutrition. *Biogerontology.* 2016;17(3):529-546. https://dspace.stir.ac.uk/bitstream/1893/22882/1/Witard%20et%20al_Biogerontology_2016.pdf

Chapter 7

Jones CJ, Rikli RE. Measuring functional fitness of older adults. *J Active Aging*. 2002;March-April:24–30. www.dsnm.univr.it/documenti/OccorrenzaIns/matdid/matdid182478.pdf. Accessed February 3, 2017.

Kenney WL, Wilmore JH, Costill DL. *Physiology of Sport and Exercise*. 6th ed. Champaign, IL: Human Kinetics; 2015.

Murray B, Kenney WL. *Practical Guide to Exercise Physiology*. Champaign, IL: Human Kinetics; 2016.

Signorile JF. *Bending the Aging Curve: The Complete Exercise Guide For Older Adults*. Champaign, IL: Human Kinetics; 2011.

Signorile JF. Targeted resistance training to improve independence and reduce fall risk in older clients. *ACSM Health Fitness J*. 2016;20(5):29-40.

Chapter 8

Davis SR, Castelo-Branco C, Chedraui P, Lumsden MA, Nappi RE, Shah D, Villeseca P. Understanding weight gain at menopause. *Climacteric*. 2012;15:419-429.

Heshmat S. *Eating Behavior and Obesity: Behavioral Economic Strategies for Health Professionals*. New York: Springer Publishing Co; 2011.

Horne BD, Muhlestein JB, Anderson JL. Health effects of intermittent fasting: hormesis or harm? A systematic review. *Am J Clin Nutr*. 2015;102(2):464-470.

Kong A, Beresford SA, Alfano CM, et al. Self-monitoring and eating-related behaviors are associated with 12-month weight loss in postmenopausal overweight-to-obese women. *J Acad Nutr Diet*. 2012;112(9):1428-1435.

Manore MM. Dietary supplements for improving body composition and reducing body weight: where is the evidence? *Int J Sport Nutr Exerc Metab*. 2012;22(2):139-154.

Michalakis K, Goulis DG, Vazaiou A, Mintziori G, Polymeris A, Abrahamian-Michalakis A. Obesity in the ageing man. *Metabolism*. 2013;62(10):1341-1349.

Navarro VJ, Khan I, Björnsson E, Seeff LB, Serrano J, Hoofnagle JH. Liver injury from herbal and dietary supplements. *Hepatology*. 2016;65(1):363-373. doi:10.1002/hep.28813

Raynor HA, Champagne CM. Position of the Academy of Nutrition and Dietetics: interventions for the treatment of overweight and obesity in adults. *J Acad Nutr Diet*. 2016;116(1):129-147.

The scam of the veggie chip. ConscienHealth website. http://conscienhealth.org/2016/04/the-scam-of-veggie-chips. Published April 10, 2016. Accessed April 10, 2016.

Tsai AC, Sandretto A, Chung YC. Dieting is more effective in reducing weight but exercise is more effective in reducing fat during the early phase of a weight-reducing program in healthy humans. *J Nutr Biochem*. 2003;14(9):541–549.

Wansink B. *Mindless Eating: Why We Eat More than We Think*. New York: Bantam Books; 2006.

Chapter 9

Brown CL, Gibbons LE, Kennison RF, et al. Social activity and cognitive functioning over time: a coordinated analysis of four longitudinal studies. *J Aging Res*. 2012;2012:287438. http://dx.doi.org/10.1155/2012/287438.
Brown TM, Fee E. Walter Bradford Cannon: pioneer physiologist of human emotions. *Am J Public Health*. 2002;92(10):1594-1595.
Byun J, Jung D. The influence of daily stress and resilience on successful aging. *Int Nurs Rev*. 2016;63(3):482-489. doi: 10.1111/inr.12297.
Chodzko-Zajko W, Proctor DN, Fiatarone Singh MA, et al. Exercise and physical activity for older adults. *Med Sci Sport Exerc*. 2009;41(7):1510-1530.
Gerst-Emerson K, Jayawardhana J. Loneliness as a public health issue: the impact of loneliness on health care utilization among older adults. *Am J Public Health*. 2015;105(5);1013-1019.
Malone JC, Cohen S, Liu SR, Vaillant GE, Waldinger RJ. Adaptive midlife defense mechanisms and late-life happiness. *Pers Individ Dif*. 2013;55:85-89.
Rowe JW, Kahn RI. Successful aging. *Gerontologist*. 1997;37(4):433-440.
Smith A. Older adults and technology use. Pew Research Center website. www.pewinternet.org/2014/04/03/older-adults-and-technology-use. Published April 3, 2014. Accessed March 12, 2017.
Steptoe A, Shankar A, Demakakos P, Wardle J. Social isolation, loneliness, and all-cause mortality in older men and women. *Proc Natl Acad Sci USA*. 2013;110(15):5797-5801.

Chapter 10

Buford TW. Hypertension and aging. *Ageing Res Rev*. 2016;26:96-111.
Cameron M, Chrubasik S. Oral herbal therapies for treating osteoarthritis. *Cochrane Database Syst Rev*. 2014;(5):CD002947. doi: 10.1002/14651858.CD002947.pub2.
Chronic diseases: the leading causes of death and disability in the United States. Centers for Disease Control and Prevention. www.cdc.gov/chronicdisease/overview/. Updated February 23, 2016. Accessed March 26, 2017.
Diagnosing diabetes and learning about prediabetes. American Diabetes Association website. www.diabetes.org/diabetes-basics/diagnosis. Updated November 21, 2016. Accessed December 20, 2016.
Diodato M, Chedrawy EG. Coronary artery bypass graft surgery: the past, present, and future of myocardial revascularization. *Surg Res Pract*. 2014;2014:1-6. doi:10.1155/2014/726158.
Federal Interagency Forum on Aging-Related Statistics. *Older Americans 2016: Key Indicators of Well-Being*. Washington, DC: US Government Printing Office; 2016. https://agingstats.gov/docs/LatestReport/Older-Americans-2016-Key-Indicators-of-WellBeing.pdf.
Heart Disease Facts. Centers for Disease Control and Prevention website. www.cdc.gov/HeartDisease/facts.htm. Updated August 10, 2015. Accessed April 2, 2017.
Lanier JB, Bury DC, Richardson SW. Diet and physical activity for cardiovascular disease prevention. *Am Fam Physician*. 2016;93(11):919-924.

Martínez-González MA, Salas-Salvadó J, Estruch R, et al. Benefits of the Mediterranean diet: insights from the PREDIMED study, *Prog Cardiovasc Dis.* 2015;58(1):50-60. doi: 10.1016/j.pcad.2015.04.003.

Messier SP, Gutekunst DJ, Davis C, DeVita P. Weight loss reduces knee-joint loads in overweight and obese older adults with knee osteoarthritis. *Arthritis Rheum.* 2005;52(7)2026-2032.

Mudryi AN, Yu N, Aukema HM. Nutritional and health benefits of pulses. *Appl Physiol Nutr Metab.* 2014;39(11):1197-1204.

Rees K, Hartley L, Flowers N, et al. “Mediterranean” dietary pattern for the primary prevention of cardiovascular disease. *Cochrane Database Syst Rev.* 2013; (8): CD009825. DOI: 10.1002/14651858.CD009825.pub2.

Sawitzke AD, Shi H, Finco MF, et al,. Clinical efficacy and safety of glucosamine, chondroitin sulphate, their combination, celecoxib or placebo taken to treat osteoarthritis of the knee: 2-year results from GAIT. *Ann Rheum Dis.* 2010;69(8):1459-1464. doi: 10.1136/ard.2009.120469.

Sharma S, Merghani A, Mont L. Exercise and the heart: the good, the bad, and the ugly. *Eur Heart J* 2015 36(23):1445-1453.

Way KL, Hackett DA, Baker MK, Johnson NA. The effect of regular exercise on insulin sensitivity in type 2 diabetes mellitus: a systematic review and meta-analysis. *Diab Metab J.* 2016;40(4):253-271.Bibliography

INDEX